Plant-Based Diet for beginners

A beginners guide to get started with plant-based diet and how to do meal plan: a strategy both useful for weight loss and well suitable for athletes

Hellen cook

Legal & Disclaimer

The information contained in this book and its contents is not designed to replace or take the place of any form of medical or professional advice; and is not meant to replace the need for independent medical, financial, legal or other professional advice or services, as may be required. The content and information in this book has been provided for educational and entertainment purposes only.

The content and information contained in this book has been compiled from sources deemed reliable, and it is accurate to the best of the Author's knowledge, information and belief. However, the Author cannot guarantee its accuracy and validity and cannot be held liable for any errors and/or omissions. Further, changes are periodically made to this book as and when needed. Where appropriate and/or necessary, you must consult a professional (including but not limited to your doctor, attorney, financial advisor or such other professional advisor) before using any of the suggested remedies, techniques, or information in this book.

Upon using the contents and information contained in this book, you agree to hold harmless the Author from and against any damages, costs, and expenses, including any legal fees potentially resulting from the application of any of the information provided by this book. This disclaimer applies to any loss, damages or injury caused by the use and application, whether directly or indirectly, of any advice or information presented, whether for breach of contract, tort, negligence, personal injury, criminal intent, or under any other cause of action.

You agree to accept all risks of using the information presented inside this book.

You agree that by continuing to read this book, where appropriate and/or necessary, you shall consult a professional (including but not limited to your doctor, attorney, or financial advisor or such other advisor as needed) before using any of the suggested remedies, techniques, or information in this book.

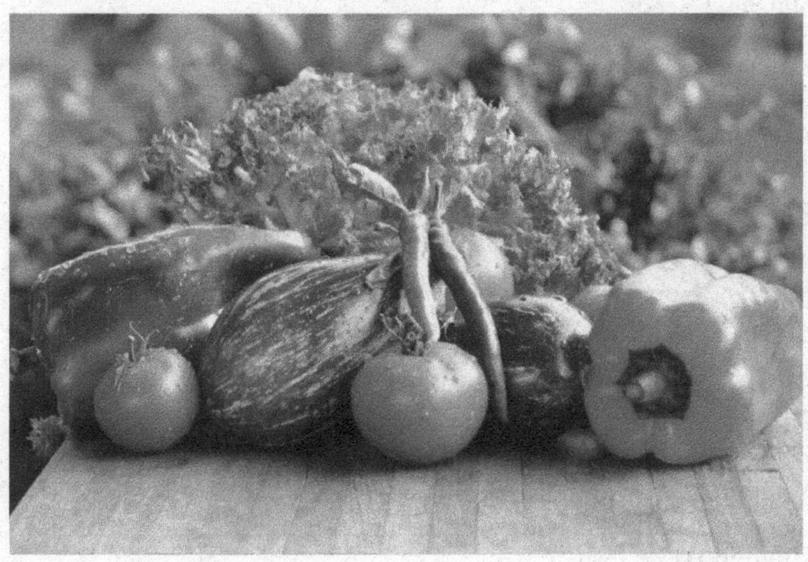

Table of Contents

Introduction

Many people believe that the only good nutrients come only from animal and without them you can't have a healthy lifestyle. What they don't understand is that the plant-based diet is a great source of nutrients needed by the body. Plants contain proteins and other nutrients found in animals. Plants have little fat in comparison to meat. The fat found in animals increases the levels of cholesterol in the body, which may increase the chances of a heart attack.

The plant-based diet is an all healthy and natural diet that comes directly from the plants and based on wholeness. The core feature of the diet is no processing involved and mixing as well. You are supposed to take the producing plants in their original form with the appropriate cooking styles and types. It is one of the major benefits that you can get all the nutrition in their original format. In the making of plant-based food options, there should not be any overcooking. The well-balanced diet with all of its natural richness brings a bundle of ultimate benefits for the consumer.

A plant-based diet is all about easy healthy plant food option that includes fruits, vegetables, lentils, beans, and more. Other than the hardcore plant diet options, it allows the intake of low-fat dairy products that includes low-fat milk, low-fat cottage, mozzarella and cheddar cheese as well. Having a plant-based diet doesn't require that you avoid all the animal-based products.

The primary focus of the plant-based whole-food diet plan is to minimize your consumption of processed foods as much as possible and replace them with more plant-based and whole natural foods proven to be beneficial in not only improving your health but also stimulating effective weight loss. Hopefully, the information in this cookbook helped clear away confusion and doubts regarding this kind of diet plan.

This book contains all information you may need to about the plant-based diet. The book also contains delicious plant-based recipes that are easy to prepare. The recipes are divided into these categories;

- Breakfast
- Lunch
- Dinner
- Soups
- Desserts and snacks
- Smoothies

Thank you for choosing this book. Enjoy reading!

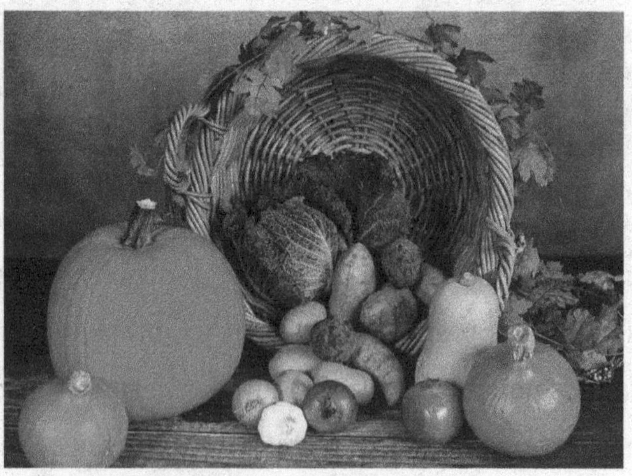

Chapter 1

History of Plant Based Diet

As you can imagine, humans have been consuming a plant-based diet before we even knew the invention of McDonald's and some of our other favorite fast-food chains. To begin our journey, I am going to start us off in the times of hunter-gatherer. While we could go back even further (think Egypt!), I believe this is where a plant-based diet becomes most relevant!

Hunting and Gathering

During this specific time in human history, the hunter-gatherer time period is where we find the earliest evidence of hunting. While we do have a long history of eating meat, this is a point in time where consuming meat was very limited. Of course, humans eating meat does not mean we were carnivores; in fact, the way we are built tells us differently. Yes, we can consume meat, but humans are considered omnivores more or less. You can tell this by our jaw design, running speeds, alimentary tract, and the fact we don't have claws attached to our fingers. With that being said, history also tells us we are omnivores by nature; however, the evolution of our human brains leads us to become hunters so that we could survive.

The need for hunting did not come around until our ancestors left tropical regions. It was in other locations that started having an effect on the availability of plant-based foods. Instead of enduring winter with limited amounts of food, we had to adapt! Of course, out of hunger, animal-flesh becomes much more appealing. This early in time, our ancestors did not have a grocery store just to pop in and buy whatever they needed. Instead, they used the opportunity of hunting and gathering to keep themselves alive.

Agriculture

Eventually, we moved away from hunting and gathering and started to become farmers! While this timeline is a bit tricky and the agriculture history began at different points in different parts of the world, all that matters is that at some point; animals started to become domesticated and dairy, eggs, and meat all became readily available. Once this started, humans no longer needed to hunt nor gather because the farmers provided everything we could desire!

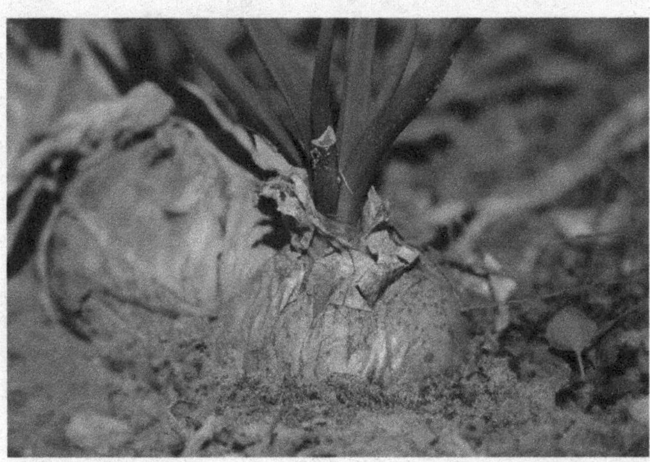

on the availability of plant-based foods instead of enduring winter with limited amounts of food we had stocked up. Of course, out of hunger and laziness becomes much more appealing. This early in time, our ancestors did not have grocery stores to pop in and buy whatever they needed. Instead, they used the opportunity of hunting and gathering to keep themselves alive.

Agriculture

Eventually, we moved away from hunting and gathering, and started to become farmers. While this happened gradually, and the agricultural history began at different points in different parts of the world, what matters is that at some point, animals started to become domesticated and dairy, eggs, and meat all became readily available. Once this started, humans no longer needed to hunt or gather because the farmers provided everything we could desire.

Chapter 2

Benefits of Plant Based Diet

While starting a plant-based diet is an excellent idea and has many wonderful benefits let's be honest, you are mostly here to benefit yourself. It is fantastic that you are deciding to put you and your health first! You deserve to be the best version of yourself, with a little bit of legwork, you will be there in no time!

To some people, a plant-based diet is just another fad diet. There are so many diets on the market right now, why is plant-based any different? Whether you are looking to lose weight, reverse disease, or just love animals; the plant-based diet can help you out in a number of different ways! On this diet, you will become healthy on the inside and healthy on the outside.

A plant-based diet is so much more than just eating fruits and vegetables. This is a lifestyle where you are encouraged to journey to a better version of yourself. As you improve your eating habits, you will need something to do with all of your new found energy! It is time to gain control over your eating habits and figure out how food truly does affect our daily lives! Below, you will find the amazing benefits a plant-based diet has to offer you.

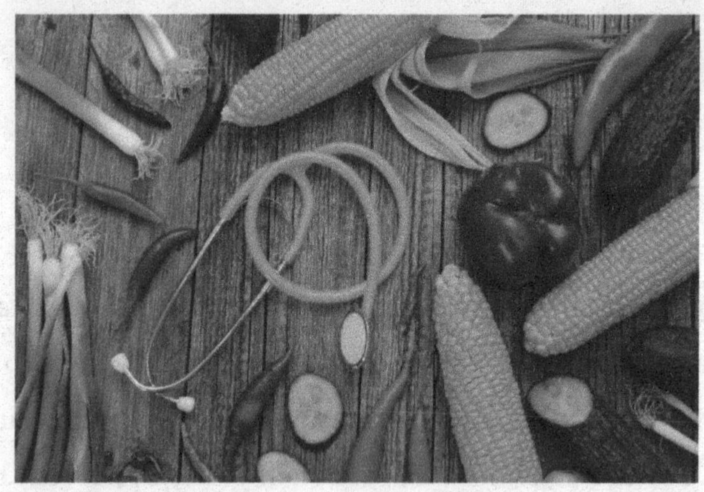

Lower Your Cholesterol

Let me start by asking you a question; how much do you think one egg affects your cholesterol? One egg a day could increase your dietary cholesterol from 97 to 418 mg in a single day! There was a study done on seventeen lacto-vegetarian college students. During this study, the students were asked to consume 400kcal in test foods along with one large egg for three weeks. During this time, their dietary cholesterol raised to these numbers. To put it in perspective, 200 to 239 mg/dL is considered borderline high.

The next question you should be asking yourself is what is considered a healthy amount of cholesterol? The answer is zero percent! There is no tolerable intake of trans fats, saturated fats, nor cholesterol. All of these (found in animal products) raise LDL cholesterol. Luckily, a plant-based diet can bring your cholesterol levels down drastically. By doing this, you will be lowering your risk of disease that is typically related to high cholesterol levels. The good news here is that your body makes the cholesterol you need! There is no need to "get it" from other sources.

Healthy Antioxidants

As of recently, there has been a push with products showing they are incredibly healthy due to the fact they contain antioxidants. These are fantastic as antioxidants help prevent the circulation of oxidized fats that are building up in your bloodstream. As you consume more antioxidants naturally in your plant-based diet, this can help reduce inflammation, lower your blood pressure, prevent blood clots, and decrease any artery stiffness you may have.

To put it into perspective, a plant can contain about sixty-four times more antioxidants compared to animal products such as meat. In the chapter to follow, you will be learning more about the foods that contain antioxidants and how to incorporate them into your diet. The good news is that these foods are healthy, natural, and delicious all at the same time!

High Fiber Intake

As you begin a plant-based diet, you will be getting more fiber in your diet naturally. You may be surprised to learn that on average, about ninety percent of Americans do not receive the proper amount of fiber! This is bad news for a majority of people as fiber has some very good benefits. Fiber has been shown to reduce the risk of stroke, obesity, heart disease, diabetes, breast cancer, and the risk of colon cancer! On top of these benefits, fiber also helps control blood sugar levels and cholesterol levels.

Asthma Benefits

According to the Centers for Disease Control and Prevention, about ten percent of children in 2009 has asthma. This means that in 2009, more children than adults had the risk of having an asthma attack. Asthma is defined as an inflammatory disease. The question is, what is causing the rise of asthma? It's all in the diet! According to one study, both eggs and sweetened beverages have been linked to asthma. On the other hand, fruits and vegetables both appear to have a positive effect on lowering asthma in children that eat at least two servings of vegetables a day. In fact, their risk of suffering from an allergic asthma attack was lowered by fifty percent!

Reduce Risk of Breast Cancer

While it can be hard to pinpoint the development of breast cancer, it seems there are three steps to creating a healthier lifestyle to lower your risk of developing it in the first place. First, you will want to maintain a normal body weight. Luckily, this can be achieved by consuming a plant-based diet. On top of eating your fruits and vegetables, you will also want to limit your alcohol consumption. By doing this, individuals have been able to reduce their risk of developing breast cancer by sixty percent! To put this into perspective, meat eaters have a seventy-four percent higher risk of developing breast cancer compared to those who eat more vegetables. I'm not sure about you, but that just doesn't seem worth it to me!

Reduce the Development of Kidney Stones

Did you know that by eating one extra can of tuna a day can increase your risk of forming a calcium stone in your urinary tract by a whopping two-hundred and fifty percent? The risk is calculated by studying the relative probability of forming a stone when high animal protein is ingested. The theory behind this is that urine needs to be more alkaline if you want to lower your risk of developing stones. When meat is consumed, this produced acid in the body. On the other hand, beans and vegetables both reduce the acid in the body, leading to a lower risk of developing kidney stones; science!

Reverse and Prevent High Blood Pressure and Heart Disease

Unfortunately, one in three Americans has high blood pressure. Studies have shown that as a diet becomes plant-based, this grants the ability to drop the rate of hypertension. In fact, there is about a seventy-five percent drop between an omnivore and a vegan! It appears as though a vegetarian diet sets a kind of protection against cardiometabolic risk factors, cardiovascular disease, as well as overall total mortality. When compared against a lacto-ovo-vegetarian diet, plant-based diets seem to also have protection against cardiovascular mortality, type-2 diabetes, hypertension, as well as obesity! This is fantastic news, especially when you lean that just three portions of whole-grain foods seem to significantly reduce the risk of cardiovascular disease in middle-aged people. This is the same benefit that a symptom-reducing drug can give you!

Control and Prevent Cancer

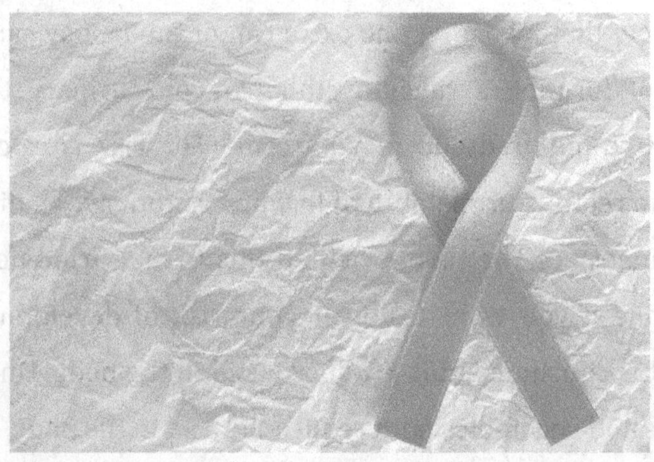

Fat from animals is often associated with the risk of developing pancreatic cancer. In fact, for every fifty grams of chicken consumed on a daily basis, your risk of developing pancreatic cancer increases by seventy-two percent! At this point in time, pancreatic cancer is the fourth most common death-causing cancer in the world. It's pretty simple to avoid if you simply switch your beef to beans!

On the other end of the spectrum, it appears that by consuming 70g of more beans a day can cut your risk of developing colon cancer by seventy-five percent. This may be due to IP which is found in cereal and beans. It appears this plays a major role in controlling tumor-growth, metastasis and preventing cancer. In addition to these benefits, IP overall seems to enhance the immune system, lower elevated serum cholesterol, prevent calcification and kidney stones, as well as reducing pathological platelet activity within the body. That seems pretty nifty for eating just a few more beans and less meat!

Decrease Insulin Resistance

Our bodies are very delicate machines. When fat begins to accumulate in your muscle cells, this interferes with insulin. When this build up happens, the insulin in the body is unable to bring the sugar out of the blood system that your body needs for energy. Unfortunately, high sugar intake makes this situation even worse and can clog your arteries altogether. When you eliminate meat from the diet, this means you will have less fat in your muscles. By decreasing these levels, you will be able to avoid insulin resistance in the first place!

Reverse and Prevent Diabetes

As of right now, diabetes is the cause of 750,000 deaths each year. Since 1990, the number of individuals in the United States diagnosed with diabetes has tripled to more than twenty million people. Within this range, you have one-hundred and thirty-two thousand children below the age of eighteen years old who suffer from diabetes. In 2014, fifty-two thousand people were diagnosed with end-age renal disease due to diabetes. Overall, the United States spent a total of two hundred and forty-five billion dollars in direct cost of diagnosing individuals with diabetes. If these numbers seem overwhelming to you, I have good news; plant-based diet can help with this issue. As you learn how to incorporate more vegetables into your diet, the risk of developing hypertension and diabetes drops by about seventy-eight percent.

Obesity Control and Weight Loss

In a study completed on various diet groups, it was shown that beans typically have a lower mass index compared to other individuals. These people were also proven to be less prone to obesity when they were compared to both vegetarians and non-vegetarians. This may be due to the fact that plant-based individuals have lower animal intake and higher fiber intake. When you reduce your caloric intake to lose weight at an unhealthy level, this has the ability to lead to unhealthy coping mechanisms such as bulimia and anorexia. As you learn how to follow a plant-based diet, you will be filling up on healthy foods such as vegetables, fruits, nuts, and whole grains. At no point on this diet should you be starving or wishing you could eat more. All of the food you will be consuming are typically low in fat and will help with weight loss.

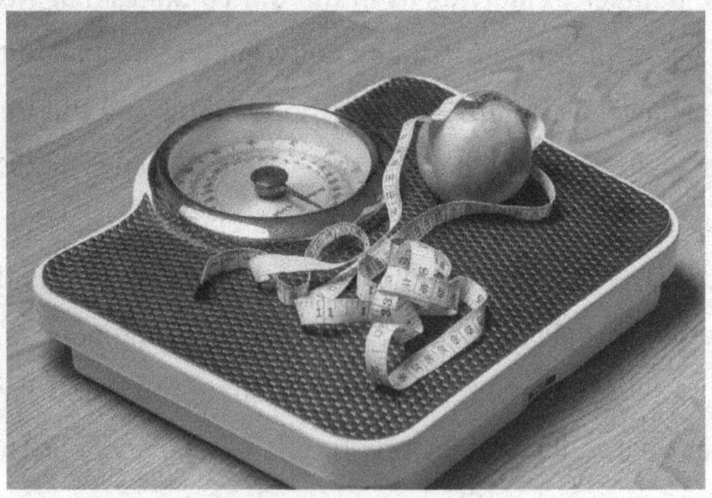

Healthier Bones

One of the common misconceptions around a plant-based diet is that due to the fact you will no longer be drinking cow's milk, you will be lacking the calcium your bones need to grow strong. While we will be going over this further in depth later, all you need to know now is that it simply is not true. While on a plant-based diet, you will be receiving plenty of essential nutrients such as vitamin K, magnesium, and potassium; all of which improve bone health.

A plant-based diet helps maintain an acid-base ratio which is very important for bone health. While on an acidic diet, this aids in the loss of calcium during urination. As you learned earlier, the more meat you consume, the more acidic your body becomes. Luckily, fruits and vegetables are high in magnesium and potassium which provides alkalinity in your diet. This means that through diet, you will be able to reduce the bone resorption.

Along the same lines, green leafy vegetables are filled with vitamin K that you need for your bones. Studies have shown that with an adequate amount of vitamin K in your diet, this can help reduce the risk of hip fractures. Along with these studies, research has also shown that soy products that have isoflavones also have a positive effect on bone health in women that are postmenopausal. By having a proper amount of isoflavones, this helps improve bone mineral density, reduce bone resorption, and helps improve overall bone formation. Overall, less calcium loss leads to reducing your risk of osteoporosis, even when calcium intake is low!

Do it for the Animals

Whether or not you are switching to a plant-based diet for reasons other than health, it never hurts to be kind and compassionate toward other sentient beings. At the end of the day, sparing someone's life is going to be the right thing to do, especially when they never asked to be brought into this world in the first place. Unfortunately, this is the whole reason behind the dairy and meat industry. In all honesty, there is nothing humane about taking lives or animal farming.

Of course, this goes beyond meat products. There are also major issues with the egg and dairy industry where dairy cows are forcefully impregnated and then have their calves taken away so we can steal their milk. These animals have feelings and emotions just like we do, what gives us the right to use them for their worth and then throw them away like garbage when we no longer have a use for them? Do the animals a favor and eat more plants, it will be better on your conscious.

Along with these same lines, you never know what is going to come with your animal products. There are a host of toxins, dioxins, hormones, antibiotics, and bacteria that can cause some serious health issues. In fact, there is a very high percentage of animal flesh that is contaminated with dangerous bacteria such as E. coli, listeria, and Campylobacter. These are all tough to find some time because these bacteria live in the flesh, feces, and intestinal tracts of the animals.

With the bacteria being tough to find and kill, this eventually can cause food poisoning. Each year, the USDA has reported that animal flesh causes about seventy percent of food poisoning per year. This means that there are about seventy-five million cases of food poisoning a year, five-thousands of which result in death.

Do it for the Environment

We were given this one planet to live on, and we should be doing everything in our power to help protect it. During these trying times, it seems that half of the population believes in climate change while the other half thinks of it as fake news. As a plant-eater, it is our duty to do our part in saving the environment. Unfortunately, the meat and farming industry is going to be a hard beast to take down. Depending on the source, it has been proven that the meat industry is behind anywhere from eighteen to fifty-one percent of man-made pollution. This puts the farm industry ahead of transportation when it comes down to the contribution of pollution to the greenhouse effect. In one pound of hamburger meat that you are consuming, this equals about seventy-five kg of CO2 emission. Do you know what produces that much CO2 emission? Three weeks from using your car! Do your part, eat more plants and save the planet.

Improve your Mood

When you are making an impact on saving the animals and saving the environment, it is no surprise that your mood will enhance! As you begin to cut back on animal products, you will be abstaining from the stress hormones those animals are producing while they are on their way to the slaughterhouse. This factor alone will have a major impact on your mood stability. By eating plants, this helps individuals lower their levels of fatigue, hostility, anger, depression, anxiety, and overall tension. The mood boost may be due to the antioxidants mentioned earlier in this chapter.

On top of these added benefits, it seems as though carbohydrate-rich foods like rye bread, steel cut oats, and brown rice all seem to have a positive effect on the serotonin levels in the brain. Serotonin is very important in controlling mood which is why a plant-based diet may help treat the symptoms that are often associated with depression and anxiety.

Skin and Digestion Improvements

You may be surprised to learn that skin and digestion are actually connected! If you suffer from acne-prone skin, dairy may be the culprit behind the issue! If you have bad acne, try a plant-based diet. As you eat more fruits and vegetables, you will be eliminating fatty foods such as oils and animal products that may be causing the acne in the first place. On top of this, fruits and vegetables are often rich in water and can provide you with high levels of minerals and vitamins. By consuming more fiber in your diet, this helps eliminate toxins in your body and boost digestion. When this happens, it could clear up your acne!

Improve Overall Fitness

Amazing things will happen as you lose weight and clean yourself from the inside out. When people first begin a plant-based diet, there is a common misconception that a lack of animal products means a lack of muscle mass and energy. Luckily, the opposite is true. It seems as though meat and dairy are both harder to digest. When these products are harder to digest, this means that it is taking more energy to do so. As you consume more fruits and vegetables on a plant-based diet, you will be amazed at how much added energy and strength you will develop.

On top of these benefits, a plant-based diet provides you with plenty of great quality proteins if you are looking to build muscle mass. While eating legumes, nuts, seeds, green vegetables, and whole grains, you will easily be consuming the forty to fifty grams of protein per day that is recommended. Of course, this number will vary but depending on your goals; you will easily be able to consume plenty of protein on a plant-based diet.

It's So Easy

When you first begin a plant-based diet, you should just expect your friends and family to doubt your life choices. You will be amazed to learn just how easy it is to live plant-based in the modern age. At the grocery store alone, there are incredible plant-based options for you and your family. There are plenty of plant-based milk options, ice creams, mock meats and more. In fact, the alternative sales in the market are expected to each about five billion dollars by 2020! Along with supermarkets, more restaurants are choosing to provide plant-based options as well. Now, you are no longer forced to cook at home if you wish to live this lifestyle. With each passing day, becoming a plant-based person is become much easier compared to earlier times.

Along with it becoming easier, it is also an economical choice. As you narrow your food choices down to seasonal fruits, vegetables, seeds, nuts, beans, and grains, you may be surprised to learn how much you will be cutting down your monthly food expenses! One of the best parts of whole foods is that you can buy them in bulk! When you purchase your foods this way, you will be spending less in a day and less on eating out.

Chapter 3

What to eat and what to avoid

Foods to eat

Now we get to the good part; eating! To start this chapter off, I first want to go over all of the food you will be able to enjoy while following a plant-based diet. There is a tremendous amount of people who like to focus on the bad when they start a diet, which is exactly why a mass majority of diets fail in the first place! Instead of focusing on what you will no longer be "allowed" to eat on your diet, it is time to learn all of the incredible foods you will be able to enjoy!

Grains

As we go through this section, I want you to imagine the food pyramid we grew up learning in school. At the very bottom of the pyramid, you will find grains; meaning that these are going to be a majority of your new diet. In fact, the recommended daily serving is about six servings of half of a cup of grains per day. As you choose grains, you will want to place a heavy emphasize on whole grains such as buckwheat, wheat berries, millet, quinoa, and brown rice.

There are other choices such as pasta, bread, and cereal but you will want to assure that these selections are as unprocessed as possible. In fact, a mass majority of your calories should come from whole starches.

You will be able to consume these foods until you are satiated! As you practice a plant-based diet, you will learn how to adjust your daily servings according to your own energy needs.

Luckily, starches are both healthy and reliable while following a plant-based diet These foods will contain a large number of complex carbohydrates which means you will stay full while getting long-lasting energy to both your brain and your body! On top of these incredible benefits, starches also provide you with minerals, fibers, essential fats, and proteins you need to improve overall health.

Whole Grains Examples

Wild Rice, Whole Grain Pasta/ Flour/ Rolls, Wheat, Spelt, Rye,

Quinoa, Millet, Farro, Corn, Buckwheat, Brown Rice, Barley,

Amaranth

Vegetables

The next tier up on the food pyramid for a plant-based diet is going to be vegetables. More than likely, you probably expected this one! For a daily recommendation, you should be striving for five or more servings of either half a cup cooked or one cup raw. In the beginning, this may seem like a difficult task, but with some extra work, every meal will include a vegetable. As you choose your vegetables, imagine that you are trying to eat the rainbow! You will be filling your plate with leafy greens and starchy root vegetables.

As you include more vegetables in your diet, you may find it difficult to eat the large bulk of the food. Remember that on a plant-based diet, it is going to be vital you receive enough calories so you can keep your energy levels up. To solve this “problem,” you can always try to consume more soups and smoothies so you can receive the proper amount of nutrients. From this point on, vegetables are going to be your new best friend!

The best part about vegetables is that they are absolute nutrient powerhouses. Vegetables are filled with the phytonutrients, antioxidants, vitamins, minerals, and fiber that your body needs in order to thrive. Whether you are eating these vegetables frozen, fresh, cooked, or raw; there are plenty of options for you to try out on a plant-based diet!

Fresh Vegetable Examples:

Zucchini, Yams, Tomatoes, Sweet Potato, Squash, Pumpkin, Onion, Mushrooms, Green Onions, Celery, Cauliflower, Carrots,

Broccoli, Bell Peppers, Asparagus, Avocado.

Leafy Green Examples:

Wheatgrass, Spring Greens, Lettuce, Kale, Bok Choy, Baby Spinach, Arugula

Fruits

Next, we have the fruit tier. Generally, you will want to eat a lower number of servings of fruits as they are generally higher in natural sugars. If you are looking to lose weight on a plant-based diet, try keeping fruit to about four servings of fruit at half of a cup per day. This way, you keep your fruit consumption in moderation. On a plant-based diet, you can choose fresh fruit, but dried food can be consumed in smaller portions. As a general note, you will want to try to avoid or limit fruit juices.

Luckily, there is a wide variety of fruits for you to choose from and you can still have them on a daily basis. Many fruits are packed with phytonutrients, antioxidants, enzymes, minerals, and the vitamins you need in order to prevent disease and feel healthier. The simple sugars in these fruits are excellent for quick energy if you want to have them as a snack.

As a general rule, you will want to consume fruit that is ripe. At this point, the fruit is both alkalizing and as nutritious as they are going to get. Fruit is wonderful and versatile as you can have them in smoothies, on your oatmeal, or all by itself. Just remember that for the best health benefits on a plant-based diet, you will still need to enjoy "nature's candy" in moderation.

Fresh Fruit Examples: Watermelon, Strawberries, Raspberries, Plums, Peaches, Oranges, Mangoes, Limes, Lemons, Cucumber, Blueberries, Bananas, Apricots

Legumes

This category will change depending on the version of the plant-based diet you choose to follow. Some dietitians say you should be eating more legumes while others say it should be limited. Cooked beans and lentils are both excellent choices and should be calcium-fortified whenever possible. This is where you are going to get a majority of your protein from. As a general rule, strive for three, half cup servings per day. Below, you will find some of the more popular versions to get you started!

Legume Examples:

White Beans, Split Peas, Snow Peas, Red Beans, Pinto Beas, Lentils, Kidney Beans, Green Beans, Chickpeas, Black Beans,

Bean Sprouts

Nuts and Seeds

Finally, we reach the top of your plant-based food pyramid! All the way up here, you will find your nuts and seeds. Being such a small portion of the pyramid, you will want to make sure that you keep these to a minimum at one-ounce servings, twice a day. This rule will need to be stricter for those of you who are looking to lose weight while following a plant-based diet.

Individuals who follow a SAD diet receive much more than the recommended 30% calories from fat; all of which are provided from saturated fats and trans fats. For this reason alone, fat generally has a terrible reputation. The truth of the matter is that unprocessed fats you receive from whole foods are healthy and help support a number of functions within the body. In fact, fats are needed to develop a properly functioning brain and nervous systems! Fat is what helps absorb vitamins and minerals into our body to ensure cell health.

Of course, everything needs to be enjoyed in moderation. There is no reason to go overboard with the fats even though it is very easy to do. It is suggested you enjoy a wide variety of healthy plant fats, so you consume the proper number of Omega-3 and Omega-6 Fatty Acids. Below, you will find some of the healthier versions to include in your diet as you go more plant-based.

Nut Examples: Walnuts, Pine Nuts, Macadamia Nuts, Hazelnuts,

Cashews, Almonds

Seed Examples: Sunflower Seeds, Pumpkin Seeds, Hemp Seeds, Flax Seeds, Chia Seeds

Critical Nutritional Needs

When you begin a plant-based diet, it will be vital that you pay special attention to the critical nutrients you need. I don't want you to look at this as a downfall because it certainly will be no issue when you are eating the proper foods, but it may be something you need to focus on when you first start. Below, we will go over some of the popular nutrients you will need and how to receive them through a plant-based diet!

Calcium

For most adults, the daily recommended intake of calcium should be about one thousand milligrams. For elderly people and teenagers, this number will be slightly more. Calcium is very important as it is needed for both nerve and muscle function. As you increase your calcium intake, you will also need an adequate amount of vitamin D in order to properly absorb the calcium into your system. Luckily, there are plenty of soy products that are fortified with calcium!

Foods Examples: Almonds, Tahini, Soy Milk, Calcium Tofu, White Beans, Navel Oranges, Kale, Broccoli, Spinach, Collard Greens

Iron

Next, iron will be a vital part of your plant-based diet. For females, the recommended amount per day is about eighteen milligrams; for females, it is only eight. Females typically need more iron during their reproductive years due to monthly blood loss. This iron is necessary for any given diet as it is in charge of transporting oxygen through the body. Iron is also beneficial for DNA synthesis and overall immune system support.

It should be noted that the iron that comes from plant sources are non-home iron, which typically isn't as well absorbed compared to the animal product iron known as home iron. What we do know is that iron from plants is safer to consume compared to the type that comes from animal products. As you increase your iron levels, you will want to add more vitamin C to enhance iron absorption. It is also beneficial to decrease coffee or tea consumption after meals, which messes with the absorption cycle.

Food Examples: Green Peas, Chickpeas, Kidney Beans, Lentils,

Dried Figs, Collard Greens, Swiss Chard, Spinach, Oatmeal, Molasses, Almonds

Zinc

Zinc is an important mineral due to the fact that it plays a major role in our immune systems and the structure of DNA. For females, the daily recommended intake is about eight and eleven if you are male. If you are a true vegan, it should be noted that the bioavailability of zinc is diminished by inhibitors in legumes, grains, and some nuts. Due to this fact, it is recommended you eat more than the recommended number so you can make sure you achieve your daily dose of zinc.

Food Examples: Almonds, Sunflower Seeds, Cashews, Pumpkin Seeds, Peas, Peanuts, Lentils, Chickpeas, Brown Rice, Oatmeal, Tofu

Iodine

For most adults, you are looking at a recommended one hundred and fifty mcg of iodine. This number will increase if you are pregnant or lactating. Iodine is very important for the production of thyroid hormones and plays a vital role in metabolism.

At this point in time, it is unclear if plant-based eaters are deficient in iodine, but it is always better to be safe than sorry! If you consume a high number of raw, cruciferous vegetables, this will be especially important as these particular foods seem to block the thyroid from absorbing iodine.

Food Examples: Iodized Salt, Seaweed, Nori, Supplement

Protein

Ah yes, the holy nutrient everyone feels you will be lacking while on a plant-based diet. As you probably could have guessed, protein is an essential macronutrient that is in charge of several important factors in the body. You have the role of maintaining bone and muscle mass, supporting the immune system, and more.

One important factor that should be noted is that the original source of all amino acids come from plant sources. On average, people typically eat way too much protein to begin with! For adults, the daily recommended intake is .8 grams per kilogram of body weight. If you are following a balanced, plant-based diet, you should have no issues consuming the proper amount of protein!

It should be noted that plant-based eaters have trouble getting lysine. To put it simply, lysine is one essential amino acid. While it is a bit harder to come by, you can find them in many of the legumes included on the plant-based diet. Below, you will find some high protein plant-based foods for you to try out!

Food Examples: Almonds, Pumpkin Seeds, Beans, Lentils, Soy Milk, Tofu, Tempeh, Whole Wheat Spaghetti, Quinoa, Seitan

Omega-3

Up to this point in your life, you have probably only gotten your omega-3 from fish. Luckily, it is possible to get these nutrients, fish-free! In fact, the essential fatty acid known as alpha-linolenic acid comes from plants and then gets converted to omega-3 within the body! This rate improves when the consumption of omega-6 is lowered so you will need to be mindful when choosing your fat sources.

Omega-3 fatty acids are important in the diet because they are linked to both brain development and heart health. The daily recommended ALA for females is about 1.1g and 1.6g for males. This number is higher for the elderly due to the fact that as we age, our bodies have a harder time converting ALA to long-chain fatty acids called DHA and EPA. Luckily, there are some easy ways to increase your omega-3 within a plant-based diet.

Food Examples: Walnuts, Hemp Seeds, Chia Seeds, Flax Seeds

Vitamin D

There are very few foods that contain vitamin D. This vitamin is a hormone that is produced in the kidneys to help the absorption of calcium. Luckily, we also get a majority of vitamin D from sunlight exposure which is why all people from plant-based to not should consider a supplement during colder and darker months.

Luckily, there are many plant-based foods that are now fortified with vitamin D. As a daily recommendation; adults should be getting fifteen mcg of vitamin D. The most reliable choice you should consider taking a supplement to assure you are getting the proper amount. Alongside with a supplement, you can also consume orange juice, cereals, and mushrooms.

Vitamin B12

Vitamin B12 is a hot topic among all plant-based diet. This is one of the only essential nutrients that is not made by plants nor animals. In fact, vitamin B12 is created by fungi and bacteria. Normally, this would be provided naturally on our foods, but though cleanliness and sterilization, all of the B12 is removed from the plant foods. The only reason people get B12 from animals is due to the fact that they are feeding on contaminated foods.

You may be surprised to learn that one-third of the population is low in B12; it doesn't matter if you are plant-based or not. If you are over the age of fifty, you should consider a supplement of B12 anyway. This is a vital vitamin to have because it plays an important role in red cell formation as well as the maintenance of the central nervous system.

Luckily, a B12 supplement is safe, easy, and cheap to buy! The daily recommendation of vitamin B12 for adults is about 2.4 mcg. Although this is recommended, it is impossible to overdose on the vitamin and should take a larger dose due to the fact that only a fraction of the supplement is absorbed. A daily dose should be about 250mcg or a weekly dose of 2500 mcg. On top of these supplements, you can also try nutritional yeast and fortified plant milk.

Foods to Avoid

A majority of the population is well aware of what plant-based individuals typically avoid on their diet. It should be noted that being plant-based is not necessarily vegan or vegetarian. Should you avoid meat? Absolutely. Is it the end of the world if you have some every once in a while? Absolutely not! Remember, you make choices for yourself. You know the health consequences of your actions, keep those choices in mind.

If you are new to plant-based, you may be surprised by some products that contain animal products, even when you think they are plant-friendly! I invite you to take a look at the list to follow so you can be aware of products that may be derived from animals. After all, there is power to knowledge!

Animal Foods

Yes, no duh! Being plant-based means that you should avoid animal foods as much as possible. Whether you are doing this for health purposes or for the love of animals, just be sure you try to avoid animal products as much as possible. Some of the more popular options include

Meat: Organs, Veal, Pork, Lamb, and Beef, etc.

Poultry: Duck, Goose, Turkey, Chicken, etc.

Eggs: Any Type of Egg

Dairy: Ice Cream, Butter, Cheese, Yogurt, etc.

Seafood and Fish: All Fish, Lobster, Crab, Mussels, Shrimp, etc.

Bee Products: Honey, Royal Jelly, etc.

Animal Derived Ingredients & Additives

This is where it can get a bit tricky when it comes to living a plant-based diet. One moment you are enjoying one of your favorite snacks, the next you are reading the label and realizing it has an ingredient that has been derived from an animal. Of course, we all make mistakes, but by being educated, you can avoid this mistake in the first place!

Dairy Ingredients: Whey, Lactose, Casein, etc.

Vitamin D3: Most vitamin D2 is derived from fish oil. You will also want to look out for lanolin which is found in sheep's wool. Instead, search from lichen, which is a vegan alternative.

Shellac: This ingredient is used for glazing sweet foods or can create a wax coating for fresh produce. Shellac is made from a female lac insect. Do yourself a favor and buy organic!

Isinglass: Do you love a good drink at the end of the day? You may want to check the label for isinglass. This is a gelatin-like substance that has been taken from the bladder of fish. Often times, it is used to help make both wine and beer.

Gelatin: This is an ingredient many people are aware of. Gelatin derives from the connective tissues, bones, and skins of cows and pigs. Be sure to read the label of any of your favorite snacks to avoid consuming gelatin.

Cochineal or Carmine: This ingredient is a natural dye that gives many foods their red color. This particular ingredient is made from ground cochineal scale insects. I am sorry to ruin different foods for you, but it is time you knew the truth and what is going into your body!

Sneaky Ingredients

As mentioned earlier, there are foods that you will think is compliant with a plant-based diet but can sometimes contain an animal-derived ingredient. For this reason, I suggest you always be cautious and check the label on everything you eat. Better yet, try to shop as fresh as possible and avoid anything with a label altogether. If it comes straight from the ground, the chances it is compliant with a plant-based diet is incredibly high.

Worcestershire Sauce: Unfortunately, there are many varieties that contain anchovies!

Dark Chocolate: A number of dark chocolates are plant-based friendly. You will want to keep an eye out for ingredients such as milk solids, nonfat milk powder, milk fat, whey, and clarified butter. All of these ingredients are animal-derived!

Roasted Peanuts: In the production of roasted peanuts, some factories use gelatin to help the salt to stick to the peanuts.

Pasta: Some pasta will contain eggs.

French Fries: When you are eating at a restaurant, you will want to be careful when it comes down to your French fries. Often times, these are fried in animal fats.

Candy: There are a wide variety of sweets that contain gelatin. Some of the more popular versions include chewing gum, gummy bears, marshmallows, and even jelly. As you can tell, these ingredients can be very sneaky!

Becoming plant-based is going to take work. The important factor is that you are making an effort to better your health and better the world around you. If you slip up a few times, do not beat yourself up! The only thing we can do is try better next time.

As you begin to navigate the plant-based world, it will become easier and easier. Every day, we are presented with multiple food choices throughout the day. If you even comply seventy-five percent of the time, you are doing better than a mass majority of the population on their SAD diet. Just remember, if it had a face and a mother, let it be!

Chapter 4

Basic Shopping List

Below is a basic plant-based shopping list:

Raisins	Walnuts	Wheatgrass
Flaxseeds	Macadamia Nuts	Spring Greens
Wild Rice	Hazelnuts	Lettuce
Wheat	Cashews	Kale
Rye	Almonds	Bok Choy
Quinoa	Sunflower Seeds	Baby Spinach
Millet	Pumpkin Seeds	Arugula
Corn	Hemp Seeds	Watermelon
Buckwheat	Snow Peas	Strawberries
Brown Rice	Red Beans	Raspberries
Barley	Pinto Beas Lentils	Plums
Amaranth	Chickpea	Peaches
Zucchini	Black Beans	Oranges
Yams	Bean Sprouts	Mangoes
Tomatoes	Broccoli	Lemons
Sweet Potato	Bell Peppers	Cucumber
Squash	Asparagus	Blueberries
Pumpkin	Avocado	Bananas
Onion	Cauliflower	Apricots

Chapter 5

Breakfast Recipes checked

Tasty Oatmeal Muffins

Prep time 10 minutes/ Cook time 20 minutes/ Serves 12

Ingredients:

- ½ cup of hot water
- ½ cup of raisins
- ¼ cup of ground flaxseed
- 2 cups of rolled oats
- ¼ teaspoon of sea salt
- ½ cup of walnuts
- ¼ teaspoon of baking soda
- 1 banana
- 2 tablespoons of cinnamon
- ¼ cup of maple syrup

Directions:

1. Whisk the flaxseed with water and allow the mixture to sit for about 5 minutes.
2. In a food processor, blend all the ingredients along with the flaxseed mix. Blend everything for 30 seconds, but do not

create a smooth substance. To create rough-textured cookies, you need to have a semi-coarse batter.

3. Put the batter in cupcake liners and place them in a muffin tin. As this is an oil-free recipe, you will need cupcake liners. Bake everything for about 20 minutes at 350 degrees.
4. Enjoy the freshly-made cookies with a glass of warm milk.

Nutritional value per serving:

Calories: 133, Fats 2 g, Carbohydrates 27 g, Protein 3 g

Omelet with Chickpea Flour

Prep time 10 minutes/ Cook time 20 minutes/ Serves 1

Ingredients:

- ½ teaspoon, onion powder
- ¼ teaspoon, black pepper
- 1 cup, chickpea flour
- ½ teaspoon, garlic powder
- ½ teaspoon, baking soda
- ¼ teaspoon, white pepper
- 1/3 cup, nutritional yeast
- 3 finely chopped green onions
- 4 ounces, sautéed mushrooms

Directions:

1. In a small bowl, mix the onion powder, white pepper, chickpea flour, garlic powder, black and white pepper, baking soda, and nutritional yeast.
2. Add 1 cup of water and create a smooth batter.
3. On medium heat, put a frying pan and add the batter just like the way you would cook pancakes.
4. On the batter, sprinkle some green onion and mushrooms. Flip the omelet and cook evenly on both sides.
5. Once both sides are cooked, serve the omelet with spinach, tomatoes, hot sauce, and salsa.

Nutritional value per serving:

Calories: 150, Fats 1.9 g, Carbohydrates 24.4 g, Proteins 10.2 g

White Sandwich Bread

Prep time 10 minutes/ Cook time 20 minutes/ Serves 16

Number of servings: 16

Ingredients:

- 1 cup warm water
- 2 tablespoons active dry yeast
- 4 tablespoons oil
- 2 ½ teaspoons salt
- 2 tablespoons raw sugar or 4 tablespoons maple syrup /agave nectar
- 1 cup warm almond milk or any other nondairy milk of your choice
- 6 cups all-purpose flour

Directions:

1. Add warm water, yeast and sugar into a bowl and stir. Set aside for 5 minutes or until lots of tiny bubbles are formed, sort of frothy.
2. Add flour and salt into a mixing bowl and stir. Pour the oil, yeast mix and milk and mix into dough. If the dough is too hard, add a little water, a tablespoon at a time and mix well each time. If the dough is too sticky, add more flour, a tablespoon at a time. Knead the dough for 8 minutes until soft and supple. You can use your hands or use the dough hook attachment of the stand mixer.

3. Now spray some water on top of the dough. Keep the bowl covered with a towel. Let it rest until it doubles in size.
4. Remove the dough from the bowl and place on your countertop. Punch the dough.
5. Line a loaf pan with parchment paper. You can also grease with some oil if you prefer. You can use 2 smaller loaf pans if you want to make smaller loaves, like I did.
6. Place the dough in the loaf pan. Now spray some more water on top of the dough. Keep the loaf pan covered with a towel. Let it rest until the dough doubles in size.
7. Bake in a preheated oven at 370° F for about 40 – 50 minutes or a toothpick when inserted in the center of the bread comes out without any particles stuck on it.
8. Let it cool to room temperature.
9. Cut into 16 equal slices and use as required. Store in a breadbox at room temperature.

Nutritional values per serving: Calories 209, Fat 4 g, Carbohydrate 35 g, Protein 1 g

A Toast to Remember

Prep time 10 minutes/ Cook time 15 minutes/ Serves 4

Ingredients:

- 1 can, black beans
- Pinch, sea salt
- 2 pieces, whole-wheat toast
- ¼ teaspoon, chipotle spice
- Pinch, black pepper
- 1 teaspoon, garlic powder
- 1 freshly juiced lime
- 1 freshly diced avocado
- ¼ cup, corn
- 3 tablespoons, finely diced onion
- ½ freshly diced tomato
- Fresh cilantro

Directions:

1. Mix the chipotle spice with the beans, salt, garlic powder, and pepper. Stir in the lime juice.
2. Boil all of these until you have a thick and starchy mix.
3. In a bowl, mix the corn, tomato, avocado, red onion, cilantro, and juice from the rest of the lime. Add some pepper and salt.
4. Toast the bread and first spread the black bean mixture followed by the avocado mix.
5. Take a bite of wholesome goodness!

Nutritional value per serving:

Calories: 290, Fats 9 g, Carbohydrates 44 g, Proteins 12 g

Tasty Panini

Prep time 5 minutes/ Cook time 0 minutes/ Serves 1

Ingredients:

- ¼ cup, hot water
- 1 tablespoon, cinnamon
- ¼ cup, raisins
- 2 teaspoons, cacao powder
- 1 ripe banana
- 2 slices, whole-grain bread
- ¼ cup, natural peanut butter

Instructions:

1. In a bowl, mix the cinnamon, hot water, raisins, and cacao powder.
2. Spread the peanut butter on the bread.
3. Cut the bananas and put them on the toast.
4. Mix the raisin mixture in a blender and spread it on the sandwich.

Nutritional value per serving:

Calories: 850, Fats 34 g, Carbohydrates 112 g, Proteins 27 g

Tasty Oatmeal and Carrot Cake

Prep time 10 minutes/ Cook time 10 minutes/ Serves 1

Ingredients:

- 1 cup, water
- ½ teaspoon, cinnamon
- 1 cup, rolled oats
- Salt
- ¼ cup, raisins
- ½ cup, shredded carrots
- 1 cup, non-dairy milk
- ¼ teaspoon, allspice
- ½ teaspoon, vanilla extract

Toppings:

- ¼ cup, chopped walnuts
- 2 tablespoons, maple syrup
- 2 tablespoons, shredded coconut

Directions:

1. Put a small pot on low heat and bring the non-dairy milk, oats, and water to a simmer.
2. Now, add the carrots, vanilla extract, raisins, salt, cinnamon and allspice. You need to simmer all of the ingredients, but do not forget to stir them. You will know that they are ready when the liquid is fully absorbed into all of the ingredients (in about 7-10 minutes).

3. Transfer the thickened dish to bowls. You can drizzle some maple syrup on top or top them with coconut or walnuts.

Nutritional value per serving:

Calories: 210, Fats 11.48 g, Carbohydrates 10.37 g, Proteins 3.8 g

Onion & Mushroom Tart with a Nice Brown Rice Crust

Prep time 10 minutes/ Cook time 55 minutes/ Serves 1

Ingredients:

- 1 ½ pounds, mushrooms, button, portabella,
- 1 cup, short-grain brown rice
- 2 ¼ cups, water
- ½ teaspoon, ground black pepper
- 2 teaspoons, herbal spice blend
- 1 sweet large onion
- 7 ounces, extra-firm tofu
- 1 cup, plain non-dairy milk
- 2 teaspoons, onion powder
- 2 teaspoons, low-sodium soy
- 1 teaspoon, molasses
- ¼ teaspoon, ground turmeric
- ¼ cup, white wine
- ¼ cup, tapioca

Directions:

1. Cook the brown rice and put it aside for later use.
2. Slice the onions into thin strips and sauté them in water until they are soft. Then, add the molasses, and cook them for a few minutes.

3. Next, sauté the mushrooms in water with the herbal spice blend. Once the mushrooms are cooked and they are soft, add the white wine or sherry. Cook everything for a few more minutes.
4. In a blender, combine milk, tofu, arrowroot, turmeric, and onion powder till you have a smooth mixture
5. On a pie plate, create a layer of rice, spreading evenly to form a crust. The rice should be warm and not cold. It will be easy to work with warm rice. You can also use a pastry roller to get an even crust. With your fingers, gently press the sides.
6. Take half of the tofu mixture and the mushrooms and spoon them over the tart dish. Smooth the level with your spoon.
7. Now, top the layer with onions followed by the tofu mixture. You can smooth the surface again with your spoon.
8. Sprinkle some black pepper on top.
9. Bake the pie at 350o F for about 45 minutes. Toward the end, you can cover it loosely with tin foil. This will help the crust to remain moist.
10. Allow the pie crust to cool down, so that you can slice it. If you are in love with vegetarian dishes, there is no way that you will not love this pie.

Nutritional value per serving:

Calories: 245.3, Fats 16.4 g, Proteins 6.8 g, Carbohydrates 18.3 g

Perfect Breakfast Shake

Prep time 5 minutes/ Cook time 0 minutes/ Serves 2

Ingredients:

- 3 tablespoons, raw cacao powder
- 1 cup, almond milk
- 2 frozen bananas
- 3 tablespoons, natural peanut butter

Directions:

1. Use a powerful blender to combine all the ingredients.
2. Process everything until you have a smooth shake.
3. Enjoy a hearty shake to kickstart your day.

Nutritional value per serving:

Calories: 330, Fats 15 g, Carbohydrates 41 g, Proteins 11 g

Beet Gazpacho

Prep time 10 minutes/ Cook time 2 minutes/ Serves 4

Ingredients:

- ½ large bunch young beets with stems, roots and leaves
- 2 small cloves garlic, peeled,
- Salt to taste
- Pepper to taste
- ½ teaspoon liquid stevia
- 1 glass coconut milk kefir
- 1 teaspoon chopped dill
- ½ tablespoon canola oil
- 1 small red onion, chopped
- 1 tablespoon apple cider vinegar
- 2 cups vegetable broth or water
- 1 tablespoon chopped chives
- 1 scallion, sliced
- Roasted baby potatoes

Directions:

1. Cut the roots and stems of the beets into small pieces. Thinly slice the beet greens.
2. Place a saucepan over medium heat. Add oil. When the oil is heated, add onion and garlic and cook until onion turns translucent.
3. Stir in the beets, roots and stem and cook for a minute.

4. Add broth, salt and water and cover with a lid. Simmer until tender.
5. Add stevia and vinegar and mix well. Taste and adjust the stevia and vinegar if required.
6. Turn off the heat. Blend with an immersion blender until smooth.
7. Place the saucepan back over it. When it begins to boil, add beet greens and cook for a minute. Turn off the heat.
8. Cool completely. Chill if desired.
9. Add rest of the ingredients and stir.
10. Serve in bowls with roasted potatoes if desired.

Nutritional values per serving:

Calories 101, Fats 5 g, Carbohydrates 14 g, Proteins 2 g

Vegetable Rice

Prep time 7 minutes/ Cook time 15 minutes/ Serves 4

Ingredients:

- ½ cup brown rice, rinsed
- 1 cup water
- ½ teaspoon dried basil
- 1 small onion, chopped
- 2 tablespoons raisins
- 5 ounces frozen peas, thawed
- ½ cup pecan halves, toasted
- 1 medium carrot, cut into matchsticks
- 4 green onions, cut into 1-inch pieces
- 1 tablespoon olive oil
- ½ teaspoon salt or to taste
- ½ teaspoon crushed red chili flakes or to taste
- Ground pepper or to taste

Directions:

1. Place a small saucepan with water over medium heat.
2. When it begins to boil, add rice and basil. Stir.
3. When it again begins to boil, lower the heat and cover with a lid. Cook for 15 minutes until all the water is absorbed and rice is cooked. Add more water if you think the rice is not cooked well.

4. Meanwhile, place a skillet over medium high heat. Add carrots, raisins and onions and sauté until the vegetables are crisp as well as tender.
5. Stir in the peas, salt, pepper and chili flakes.
6. Add pecans and rice and stir.
7. Serve.

Nutritional values per serving:

Calories 305, Fats 13 g, Carbohydrates 41 g, Proteins 8 g

Courgette Risotto

Prep time 10 minutes/ Cook time 5 minutes/ Serves 8

Ingredients:

- 2 tablespoons olive oil
- 4 cloves garlic, finely chopped
- 1.5 pounds Arborio rice
- 6 tomatoes, chopped
- 2 teaspoons chopped rosemary
- 6 courgettes, finely diced
- 1 ¼ cups peas, fresh or frozen
- 12 cups hot vegetable stock
- 1 cup chopped
- Salt to taste
- Freshly ground pepper

Directions:

1. Place a large heavy bottomed pan over medium heat. Add oil. When the oil is heated, add onion and sauté until translucent.
2. Stir in the tomatoes and cook until soft.
3. Next stir in the rice and rosemary. Mix well.
4. Add half the stock and cook until dry. Stir frequently.
5. Add remaining stock and cook for 3-4 minutes.
6. Add courgette and peas and cook until rice is tender. Add salt and pepper to taste.
7. Stir in the basil. Let it sit for 5 minutes.

Nutritional values per serving:

Calories 406, Fats 5 g, Carbohydrates 82 g, Proteins 14 g

Chapter 6

Lunch Recipes

Brown Basmati Rice Pilaf

Prep time 10 minutes/ Cook time 3 minutes/ Serves 2

Ingredients:

- ½ tablespoon vegan butter
- ½ cup mushrooms, chopped
- ½ cup brown basmati rice
- 2-3 tablespoons water
- 1/8 teaspoon dried thyme
- Ground pepper to taste
- ½ tablespoon olive oil
- ¼ cup green onion, chopped
- 1 cup vegetable broth
- ¼ teaspoon salt
- ¼ cup chopped, toasted pecans

Directions:

1. Place a saucepan over medium-low heat. Add butter and oil.
2. When it melts, add mushrooms and cook until slightly tender.
3. Stir in the green onion and brown rice. Cook for 3 minutes. Stir constantly.

4. Stir in the broth, water, salt and thyme.
5. When it begins to boil, lower heat and cover with a lid. Simmer until rice is cooked. Add more water or broth if required.
6. Stir in the pecans and pepper.
7. Serve.

Nutritional value per serving:

Calories 189, Fats 11 g, Carbohydrates 19 g, Proteins 4 g

Mexican Rice

Prep time 10 minutes/ Cook time 15 minutes/ Serves 4

Ingredients:

- ½ can diced tomatoes with its liquid
- 2 ounces corn
- ½ can tomatoes with green chilies with its liquid
- 1 small onion, chopped
- ½ can black beans, drained, rinsed
- 1 small green bell pepper, chopped
- 1 tablespoon olive oil
- ½ cup white rice
- ¾ cup water
- 2 -3 tablespoons picante style salsa
- 2 tablespoons black olives, pitted, sliced
- 1 jalapeno pepper, sliced
- Vegan sour cream to serve
- Vegan cheese, shredded to serve

Directions:

1. Place a pan over medium heat. Add oil. When the oil is heated, add bell pepper and onions and sauté until tender.
2. Add rest of the ingredients except vegan sour cream and cheese. Stir and bring to the boil.
3. Lower the heat. Cover and cook for 15 minutes until rice is tender.

4. Serve garnished with vegan sour cream and cheese.

Nutritional values per serving:

Calories 133.8, Fats 0.7 g, Carbohydrates 27.5 g, Proteins 6.1 g

Artichoke & Eggplant Rice

Prep time 5 minutes/ Cook time 10 minutes/ Serves 3

Ingredients:

- 2 tablespoons olive oil
- 1 medium onion, finely chopped
- A handful parsley, chopped
- 1 teaspoon turmeric powder
- 3 cups vegetable stock
- Juice, lemon
- 1 eggplant, chopped into chunks
- 1 clove garlic, crushed
- 1 teaspoon smoked paprika
- 7 ounces paella rice
- 1 package chargrilled artichoke
- Lemon wedges to serve

Directions:

1. Place a nonstick pan or paella pan over medium heat. Add 1 tablespoon oil. When the oil is heated, add eggplant and cook until brown all over.
2. Remove with a slotted spoon and place on a plate lined with paper towels.
3. Add 1 tablespoon oil. When the oil is heated, add onion and sauté until translucent.

4. Stir in garlic and parsley stalks. Cook for 10 minutes. Add all the spices and rice and stir-fry for a few minutes until rice is well coated with the oil.
5. Add salt and mix well. Pour half the broth and cook until dry. Stir occasionally.
6. Add eggplant and artichokes and stir. Pour remaining stock and cook until rice is tender. Add parsley leaves and lemon juice and stir.
7. Serve hot with lemon wedges.

Nutritional values per serving:

Calories 431, Fats 16 g, Carbohydrates 58 g, Proteins 8 g

Black Beans and Rice

Prep time 6 minutes/ Cook time 15 minutes/ Serves 3

Ingredients:

- 1 tablespoon vegetable oil
- ½ can
- 1 ½ teaspoons dried oregano
- ½ cup uncooked rice
- 1 large onion, chopped
- ¼ teaspoon creole seasoning
- ¼ teaspoon ground cumin
- ¾ teaspoon garlic powder
- ½ teaspoon salt or to taste
- 1 cup water
- Cilantro to garnish

Directions:

1. Place a saucepan over medium heat. Add oil. When the oil is heated, add onions and sauté until tender. Add rest of the ingredients except rice and beans and mix well.
2. When it begins to boil, add rice and mix well.
3. Lower the heat and cover with a lid. Simmer for 15 minutes until rice is tender.
4. Turn off the heat. Let it sit covered for 5 minutes.
5. Fluff with a fork. Add beans and stir. Cover and let it sit for 5 minutes.
6. Garnish with cilantro if desired and serve.

Nutritional values per serving:

Calories 233, Fats 5 g, Carbohydrates 39.9 g, Proteins 7 g

Artichoke White Bean Sandwich Spread

Prep time 10 minutes/ Cook time 0 minutes/ Serves 4

Ingredients:

- ½ cup raw cashews, chopped
- Water
- 1 clove garlic, cut into half
- 1 tablespoon lemon zest
- 1 teaspoon fresh rosemary, chopped
- ¼ teaspoon salt
- ¼ teaspoon pepper
- 6 tablespoons almond
- 1 15.5-ounce can cannellini beans, rinsed and drained well
- 3 to 4 canned artichoke hearts, chopped
- ¼ cup hulled sunflower seeds
- Green onions, chopped, for garnish

Directions:

1. Soak the raw cashews for 15 minutes in enough water to cover them. Drain and dab with a paper towel to make them as dry as possible.
2. Transfer the cashews to a blender and add the garlic, lemon zest, rosemary, salt and pepper. Pulse to break everything up and then add the milk, one tablespoon at a time, until the mixture is smooth and creamy.

3. Mash the beans in a bowl with a fork. Add the artichoke hearts and sunflower seeds. Toss to mix.
4. Pour the cashew mixture on top and season with more salt and pepper if desired. Mix the ingredients well and spread on whole-wheat bread, crackers, or a wrap.

Nutritional values per serving:

Calories 200, Fats 4 g, Carbohydrates 39 g, Proteins 8 g

Buffalo Chickpea Wraps

Prep time 10 minutes/ Cook time 5 minutes/ Serves 3

Ingredients:

- ¼ cup plus 2 tablespoons hummus
- 2 tablespoons lemon juice
- 1½ tablespoons maple syrup
- 1 to 2 tablespoons hot water
- 1 head Romaine lettuce, chopped
- 1 15-ounce can chickpeas, drained, rinsed and patted dry
- 4 tablespoons hot sauce, divided
- 1 tablespoon olive or coconut oil
- ¼ teaspoon garlic powder
- 1 pinch sea salt
- 4 wheat tortillas
- ¼ cup cherry tomatoes, diced
- ¼ cup red onion, diced
- ¼ ripe avocado, thinly sliced

Directions:

1. Mix the hummus with the lemon juice and maple syrup in a large bowl. Use a whisk and add the hot water, a little at a time until it is thick but spreadable.
2. Add the Romaine lettuce and toss to coat. Set aside.

3. Pour the prepared chickpeas into another bowl. Add three tablespoons of the hot sauce, the olive oil, garlic powder and salt; toss to coat.
4. Heat a metal skillet (cast iron works the best) over medium heat and add the chickpea mixture. Sauté for three to five minutes and mash gently with a spoon.
5. Once the chickpea mixture is slightly dried out, remove from the heat and add the rest of the hot sauce. Stir it in well and set aside.
6. Lay the tortillas on a clean, flat surface and spread a quarter cup of the buffalo chickpeas on top. Top with tomatoes, onion and avocado and wrap.

Nutritional values per serving:

Calories 207, Fats 5 g, Carbohydrates 9 g, Proteins 8 g

Coconut Veggie Wraps

Prep time 8 minutes/ Cook time 0 minutes/ Serves 3

Ingredients:

- 1½ cups shredded carrots
- 1 red bell pepper, seeded and thinly sliced
- 2½ cups kale
- 1 ripe avocado, thinly sliced
- 1 cup fresh cilantro, chopped
- 5 coconut wraps
- 2/3 cups hummus
- 6½ cups green curry paste

Directions:

1. Slice, chop and shred all the vegetables.
2. Lay a coconut wrap on a clean flat surface and spread two tablespoons of the hummus and one tablespoon of the green curry paste on top of the end closest to you.
3. Place some carrots, bell pepper, kale and cilantro on the wrap and start rolling it up, starting from the edge closest to you. Roll tightly and fold in the ends.
4. Place the wrap, seam down, on a plate to serve.

Nutritional values per serving:

Calories 304, Fats 6 g, Carbohydrates 30 g, Proteins 4 g

Cucumber Avocado Sandwich

Prep time 5 minutes/ Cook time 10 minutes/ Serves 2

Ingredients:

- ½ of a large cucumber, peeled, sliced
- ¼ teaspoon salt
- 4 slices whole-wheat bread
- 4 ounces goat cheese with or without herbs
- 2 Romaine lettuce leaves
- 1 large avocado, peeled, pitted, sliced
- 2 pinches lemon pepper
- 1 squeeze of lemon juice
- ½ cup alfalfa sprouts

Directions:

1. Peel and slice the cucumber thinly. Lay the slices on a plate and sprinkle them with a quarter to a half teaspoon of salt. Let this set for 10 minutes or until water appears on the plate.
2. Place the cucumber slices in a colander and rinse with cold water. Let this drain, then place on a dry plate and pat dry with a paper towel.
3. Spread all slices with goat cheese and place lettuce leaves on the two bottom pieces of bread.
4. Layer the cucumber slices and avocado atop the bread.
5. Sprinkle one pinch of lemon pepper over each sandwich and drizzle a little lemon juice over the top.

6. Top with the alfalfa sprouts and place another piece of bread, goat cheese down, on top.

Nutritional values per serving:

Calories 246, Fats 3 g, Carbohydrates 19 g, Proteins 6 g

Lentil Sandwich Spread

Prep time 10 minutes/ Cook time 18 minutes/ Serves 3

Ingredients:

- 1 tablespoon water or oil
- 1 small onion, chopped
- 2 cloves garlic, minced
- 1 cup dry lentils
- 2 cups vegetable stock
- 1 tablespoon apple cider vinegar
- 2 tablespoons tomato paste
- 3 sun-dried tomatoes
- 2 tablespoons maple or agave syrup
- 1 teaspoon dried oregano
- ½ teaspoon ground cumin
- 1 teaspoon coriander
- 1 teaspoon turmeric
- ½ lemon, juiced
- 1 tablespoon fresh parsley, chopped

Directions:

1. Warm a Dutch oven over medium heat and add the water or oil.
2. Immediately add the onions and sauté for two to three minutes or until softened. Add more water if this starts to stick to the pan.
3. Add the garlic and sauté for one minute.

4. Add the lentils, vegetable stock and vinegar; bring to a boil. Turn down to a simmer and cook for 15 minutes or until the lentils are soft and the liquid is almost completely absorbed.
5. Ladle the lentils into a food processor and add the tomato paste, sun-dried tomatoes and syrup; process until smooth.
6. Add the oregano, cumin, coriander, turmeric and lemon; processes until thoroughly mixed.
7. Remove the spread to a bowl and apply it to bread, toast, a wrap, or pita. Sprinkle With toppings as desired.

Nutritional values per serving:

Calories 300, Fats 6 g, Carbohydrates 32 g, Proteins 4 g

Mediterranean Tortilla Pinwheels

Prep time 3 minutes/ Cook time 0 minutes/ Serves 2

Ingredients:

- ½ cup water
- 4 tablespoons white vinegar
- 3 tablespoons lemon juice
- 3 tablespoons tahini paste
- 1 clove garlic, minced
- Salt and pepper to taste
- Canned artichokes, drained, thinly sliced
- Cherry tomatoes, thinly sliced
- Olives, thinly sliced
- Lettuce or baby spinach
- Tortillas

Directions:

1. In a bowl, combine the water, vinegar, lemon juice and Tahini paste; whisk together until smooth.
2. Add the garlic, salt and pepper to taste; whisk to combine. Set the bowl aside.
3. Lay a tortilla on a flat surface and spread with one tablespoon of the sauce.
4. Lay some lettuce or spinach slices on top, then scatter some artichoke, tomato and olive slices on top.

5. Tightly roll the tortilla and fold in the sides. Cut the ends off and then slice into four or five pinwheels.

Nutritional values per serving:

Calories 290, Fats 6 g, Carbohydrates 24 g, Proteins 8 g

Pita Pizza

Prep time 3 minutes/ Cook time 10 minutes/ Serves 2

Ingredients:

- 1 pita
- Hummus
- Marinara sauce
- Various chopped vegetables, onions, cauliflower, broccoli, mushrooms etc.
- Shredded cheese, regular or vegan

Directions:

1. Preheat the oven to 350 degrees, Fahrenheit.
2. Place the pita bread on a baking pan coated with nonstick spray.
3. Spread the pita with hummus and then spoon on a light layer of marinara sauce.
4. Lay down your vegetables on top and sprinkle with cheese.
5. Bake for five to 10 minutes until everything is hot and bubbly.

Nutritional values per serving:

Calories 176, Fats 5 g, Carbohydrates 3 g, Proteins 6 g

Rice and Bean Burritos

Prep time 5 minutes/ Cook time 15 minutes/ Serves 4

Ingredients:

- 2 16-ounce cans fat-free refried beans
- 6 tortillas
- 2 cups cooked rice
- ½ cup salsa
- 1 tablespoon olive oil
- 1 bunch green onions, chopped
- 2 bell peppers, finely chopped
- Guacamole

Directions:

1. Preheat the oven to 375 degrees, Fahrenheit.
2. Dump the refried beans into a saucepan and place over medium heat to warm.
3. Heat the tortillas and lay them out on a flat surface.
4. Spoon the beans in a long mound that runs across the tortilla, just a little off from center.
5. Spoon some rice and salsa over the beans; add the green pepper and onions to taste, along with any other finely chopped vegetables you like.
6. Fold over the shortest edge of plain tortilla and roll it up, folding in the sides as you go.

7. Place each burrito, seam side down, on a nonstick-sprayed baking sheet.
8. Brush with olive oil and bake for 15 minutes.
9. Serve with guacamole.

Nutritional values per serving:

Calories 164, Fats 5 g, Carbohydrates 23 g, Proteins 2 g

Ricotta Basil Pinwheels

Prep time 5 minutes/ Cook time 0 minutes/ Serves 3

Ingredients:

- ½ cup unsalted cashews
- Water
- 7 ounces firm tofu, cut into pieces
- ¼ cup almond milk
- 1 teaspoon white wine vinegar
- 1 clove garlic, smashed
- 20 to 25 fresh basil leaves
- Salt and pepper to taste
- 8 tortillas
- 7 ounces fresh spinach
- ½ cup black olives, sliced
- 2 to 3 tomatoes, cut into small pieces

Directions:

1. Soak the cashews for 30 minutes in enough water to cover them. Drain them well and pat them dry with paper towels.
2. Place the cashews in a blender along with the tofu, almond milk, vinegar, garlic, basil leaves, salt and pepper to taste. Blend until smooth and creamy.
3. Spread the resulting mixture on the eight tortillas, dividing it equally.
4. Top with spinach leaves, olives and tomatoes.

5. Tightly roll each loaded tortilla.
6. Cut off the ends with a sharp knife and slice into four or five pinwheels.

Nutritional values per serving:

Calories 290, Fats 3 g, Carbohydrates 19 g, Proteins 4 g

Sloppy Joes Made with Lentils and Bulgur

Prep time 5 minutes/ Cook time 35 minutes/ Serves 6

Ingredients:

- 5 tablespoons vegetable stock
- 2 stalks celery, diced
- 1 small onion, diced
- 1 small red bell pepper, diced
- 1 teaspoon garlic powder
- 1 teaspoon chili powder
- 1 teaspoon ground cumin
- 1 teaspoon salt
- 1 cup cooked bulgur wheat
- 1 cup red lentils
- 1 15-ounce can tomato sauce
- 4 tablespoons tomato paste
- 3½ cups water
- 2 teaspoons balsamic vinegar
- 1 tablespoon Hoisin sauce

Directions:

1. In a Dutch oven, heat up the vegetable stock and add the celery, onion and bell pepper. Sauté until vegetables are soft, about five minutes.
2. Add the garlic powder, chili powder, cumin and salt and mix in.

3. Add the bulgur wheat, lentils, tomato sauce, tomato paste, water, vinegar and Hoisin sauce. Stir and bring to a boil.
4. Turn the heat down to a simmer and cook uncovered for 30 minutes. Stir occasionally to prevent sticking and scorching.
5. Taste to see if the lentils are tender.
6. When the lentils are done, serve on buns.

Nutritional values per serving:

Calories 103, Fats 4 g, Carbohydrates 3 g, Proteins 2 g

Spicy Hummus and Apple Wrap

Prep time 7 minutes/ Cook time 0 minutes/ Serves 3

Ingredients:

- 3 to 4 tablespoons hummus
- 2 tablespoons mild salsa
- ½ cup broccoli slaw
- ½ teaspoon fresh lemon juice
- 2 teaspoons plain yogurt
- salt and pepper to taste
- 1 tortilla
- Lettuce leaves
- ½ Granny Smith, cored and thinly sliced

Directions:

1. In a small bowl, mix the hummus with the salsa. Set the bowl aside.
2. In a large bowl, mix the broccoli slaw, lemon juice and yogurt. Season with the salt and pepper.
3. Lay the tortilla on a flat surface and spread on the hummus mixture.
4. Lay down some lettuce leaves on top of the hummus.
5. On the upper half of the tortilla, place a pile of the broccoli slaw mixture and cover with the apples.
6. Fold and wrap.

Nutritional values per serving:

Calories 204, Fats 10 g, Carbohydrates 49 g, Proteins 5 g

Sun-dried Tomato Spread

Prep time 10 minutes/ Cook time 0 minutes/ Serves 4

Ingredients:

- 1 cup sun-dried tomatoes
- 1 cup raw cashews
- Water for soaking tomatoes and cashews
- ½ cup water
- 1 clove garlic, minced
- 1 green onion, chopped
- 5 large basil leaves
- ½ teaspoon lemon juice
- ¼ teaspoon salt
- 1 dash pepper
- Hulled sunflower seeds, salted or unsalted

Directions:

1. Soak tomatoes and cashews for 30 minutes in separate bowls, with enough water to cover them. Drain and pat dry.
2. Put the tomatoes and cashews in a food processor and puree them, drizzling the water in as it purees to make a smooth, creamy paste.
3. Add the garlic, onion, basil leaves, lemon juice, salt and pepper and mix thoroughly.
4. Scrape into a bowl, cover and refrigerate overnight.

5. Spread on bread or toast and sprinkle with sunflower seeds for a little added crunch.

Nutritional values per serving:

Calories 123, Fats 4 g, Carbohydrates 10 g, Proteins 8 g

Sweet Potato Sandwich Spread

Prep time 10 minutes/ Cook time 0 minutes/ Serves 5

Ingredients:

- 1 large sweet potato baked and peeled
- 1 teaspoon cumin
- 1 teaspoon chili powder
- 1 teaspoon garlic powder
- Salt and pepper to taste
- 2 slices whole-wheat bread
- 1 to 2 tablespoons pinto beans, drained
- Lettuce

Directions:

1. Bake and peel the sweet potato and mash it in a bowl. If it is too thick, add a little almond or coconut milk.
2. Mix in the cumin, chili powder, garlic powder, salt and pepper.
3. Spread the mixture on a slice of bread and spoon some beans on top.
4. Top with lettuce leaves and the other slice of bread.

Nutritional values per serving:

Calories 102, Fats 3 g, Carbohydrates 4 g, Proteins 8 g

Zucchini Sandwich with Balsamic Dressing

Prep time 5 minutes/ Cook time 3 minutes/ Serves 4

Ingredients:

- 2 small zucchinis
- 1 tablespoon olive oil
- 4 cloves garlic, thinly sliced
- 1 tablespoon balsamic vinegar
- 1 large roasted red pepper, chopped
- 1 cup cannellini beans, rinsed, drained
- 2 whole-wheat sandwich rolls
- 6 to 8 basil leaves
- ½ teaspoon pepper

Directions:

1. Add the oil to a hot skillet and sauté the garlic for one or two minutes or until it just starts to brown.
2. Add the zucchini strips and sauté in batches and lay out on a plate until they are all finished.
3. Reduce heat to medium and place all the zucchini strips back in the pan.
4. Add the vinegar and sauté for about a minute.
5. In the blender, process the red pepper and beans until smooth.
6. Toast the buns and spoon onto the bottom halves the bean and pepper mixture.
7. Lay basil leaves on top and then the zucchini.

8. Grind some pepper on top and close the sandwich with the top of the bun.
9. The next chapter will give you some salads that can also make a great lunch.

Nutritional values per serving:

Calories 100, Fats 7 g, Carbohydrates 19 g, Proteins 5 g

Apple Mint Salad With Pine Nut Crunch

Prep time 10 minutes/ Cook time 0 minutes/ Serves 2

Ingredients:

- 1 medium apple, diced
- 1 tablespoon lemon juice
- 1 teaspoon maple syrup
- ½ teaspoon dried mint
- 1 tablespoon fresh pomegranate seeds
- 1 teaspoon pine nuts or sliced almonds

Directions:

1. Toast the nuts in a pan on the stove. Stir constantly so they don't burn and let them turn a golden brown. Set the pan aside until cooled to room temperature.
2. Place the diced apple in a small bowl with the lemon juice and stir around so all the apple is coated.
3. Add the maple syrup and dried mint and stir it in.
4. Sprinkle the top of the salad with pomegranate seeds and toasted nuts.

Nutritional values per serving:

Calories 104, Fats 5 g, Carbohydrates 4 g, Proteins 6 g

Chickpea 'N Spinach Tomato Salad

Prep time 7 minutes/ Cook time 0 minutes/ Serves 2

Ingredients:

- 2 cups canned or cooked chickpeas
- 4 medium tomatoes, chopped
- 5 green onions, chopped
- 1 red bell pepper, seeded,chopped
- 1/3 cup fresh parsley, chopped
- 1 cup baby spinach leaves
- 2 tablespoons olive oil
- ½ lemon, juiced
- 1 tablespoon balsamic vinegar
- 2 tablespoons flaxseed
- 2 tablespoons sesame seeds

Directions:

1. Combine the chickpeas, tomatoes, onion, bell pepper, parsley and baby spinach in a large salad bowl.
2. In a jar with a lid, combine the oil, lemon juice and balsamic vinegar; shake until well mixed.
3. Pour the dressing over the salad and sprinkle with the flaxseed and sesame seeds.

Nutritional values per serving:

Calories 165, Fats 5 g, Carbohydrates 4 g, Proteins 7 g

Mango and Red Cabbage Slaw

Prep time 15 minutes/ Cook time 0 minutes/ Serves 5

Ingredients:

- 2 ripe mangos, sliced
- ¼ cup fresh cilantro, chopped
- 4 carrots, peeled and grated
- 4 cups red cabbage, shredded
- 1 splash of balsamic vinegar
- 1 lime, juiced
- 1 pinch kosher salt

Directions:

1. Place the mango, cilantro, carrot and red cabbage in a large salad bowl.
2. Whisk together in another bowl the vinegar, lime juice and salt.
3. Pour the dressing over the salad and toss to coat.
4. For the most refreshing flavor, refrigerate for 20 minutes before serving.

Nutritional values per serving:

Calories 100, Fats 5 g, Carbohydrates 19 g, Proteins 4 g

Chapter 7

Soups Recipes

Sniffle Soup

Prep time 5 minutes/ Cook time 33 minutes/ Serves 6

Ingredients:

- 1½ tbsp plus 4 cups water, divided
- 1½ cups onion, diced
- 1 cup carrot, diced
- 1 cup celery, diced
- 3 large cloves garlic, minced
- 1 tsp paprika
- 1 tsp mild curry powder
- ½ tsp sea salt
- ¼ tsp dried thyme
- Freshly ground black pepper
- 2 cups dried red lentils
- 3 cups vegetable stock
- 1½ tbsp apple cider vinegar

Directions:

1. Heat a large pot over medium heat.
2. Add all ingredients to the pot and stir occasionally.

3. Cook for 8 minutes.
4. Increase heat and bring it to a boil.
5. Once it is boiled, let it simmer for 25 minutes.
6. Serve and enjoy.

Nutritional values per serving:

Calories 290, Fat 0.9 g, Carbs 52.7 g, Protein 18.3 g

French Lentil Soup with Paprika

Prep time 10 minutes/ Cook time 43 minutes/ Serves 5

Ingredients:

- Splash water
- 1½ cups onion, diced
- 1 cup carrot, cut into disks
- 4- 5 cloves garlic, minced
- 1½ tsp dried thyme
- 1¼ to 1½ tsp smoked paprika
- 1 tsp Dijon mustard
- ¾ tsp sea salt
- Freshly ground black pepper
- 2 cups French lentils, rinsed
- 2 cups vegan vegetable stock
- 5 cups water
- ¼ cup tomato paste
- 1 bay leaf

Directions:

1. Heat a large pot over medium heat.
2. Add all ingredients in it to the pot and cook for 8 minutes, stirring occasionally.
3. Increase heat and bring it to a boil.
4. Once it is boiled, let it simmer for 35 minutes.
5. Remove bay leaf.
6. Serve and enjoy.

Nutritional values per serving:

Calories 109, Fat 0.9 g, Carbs 26.1 g, Protein 5.7 g

Squash Soup

Prep time 10 minutes/ Cook time 1 hour 5 minutes/ Serves 4

Ingredients:

- 3 lb. butternut squash or other deep orange winter squash, whole and unpeeled
- 1 large or 2 small onions, whole and unpeeled
- 2 cups water plus more to thin
- ½ cup raw cashews, presoaked and drained
- 1 tbsp lemon juice, freshly squeezed
- 1 tsp fresh rosemary
- 1 tsp sea salt
- ¼ tsp cinnamon
- 1/8 tsp allspice
- 1 medium-large clove garlic, minced

Directions:

1. Preheat oven to 450 F.
2. Take a baking dish and line it with parchment paper.
3. Place onion and squash on the baking dish and bake for an hour.
4. Take a blender and add water, cashews, lemon juice, rosemary, sea salt, cinnamon, allspice, and garlic.
5. Puree until smooth.
6. Chop baked onions and squash and transfer to the blender with the skin and seeds removed.
7. Blend until smooth.

8. Transfer the soup to a pot and heat over low heat for 3 to 5 minutes and serve.

Nutritional values per serving:

Calories 125, Fat 8.2 g, Carbs 11.4 g, Protein 3.7 g

Chickpea Lentil Soup

Prep time 10 minutes/ Cook time 31 minutes/ Serves 6

Ingredients:

- Water
- 2 cups onion, diced
- ¾ tsp sea salt
- Freshly ground black pepper
- 1 tsp mustard seeds
- 1 tsp cumin seeds
- 1½ tsp paprika
- ½ tsp dried oregano
- ½ tsp dried thyme
- 1 cup dried red lentils
- 3½ cups chickpeas, cooked
- 2 cups tomatoes, chopped
- 3 cups vegetable stock
- 2 cups water
- 2 dried bay leaves
- ¼ cup fresh lemon juice

Directions:

1. Heat a large pot over medium heat.
2. Add all ingredients to it and cook for 6 minutes, stirring occasionally.
3. Increase heat and bring it to a boil.
4. Once it is boiled, let it simmer for 25 minutes.
5. Remove bay leaf.
6. Serve and enjoy.

Nutritional values per serving:

Calories 578, Fat 9 g, Carbs 98 g, Protein 32.1 g

Beans and Lentils Soup

Prep time 10 minutes/ Cook time 48 minutes/ Serves 4

Ingredients:

- 2 tbsp water
- 1½ cups onion, diced
- 3 cups potatoes, cut in chunks
- ½ cup celery, diced
- 1 cup carrots, diced
- 4-5 cloves garlic, minced
- 1½ tsp dried rosemary leaves
- 1 tsp dried thyme leaves
- 1½ tsp ground mustard
- 1 tsp sea salt
- Freshly ground black pepper
- 1 cup green lentils, rinsed
- 2 cups vegetable stock
- 5 cups water
- 1 tbsp red miso
- 1½ tbsp blackstrap molasses
- 2 dried bay leaves
- 15-oz can white beans

Directions:

1. Heat a large pot over medium heat.

2. Add all ingredients to it and cook for 8 minutes, stirring occasionally.
3. Increase heat and bring it to a boil.
4. Once it is boiled, let it cook for 40 minutes.
5. Remove bay leaf.
6. Serve and enjoy.

Nutritional values per serving:

Calories 292, Carbs 61.7 g, Fat 2.3 g, Protein 13.7 g

Calories 200, Fats 4 g, Carbohydrates 39 g, Proteins 8 g

Barley Lentil Stew

Prep time 5 minutes/ Cook time 50 minutes/ Serves 3

Ingredients:

- ½ onion, chopped
- 2 stalks celery, chopped
- 1 carrot, diced
- 1 tablespoon olive oil
- 3 cups vegetable stock
- 2 small red potatoes, skin on, chopped
- ¼ cup dry, uncooked barley
- ¾ cup cooked lentils

Directions:

1. Place a large pot over medium high heat and add the oil. Once it is heated, add the vegetables and sauté for three to four minutes, until slightly softened.
2. Add the vegetable stock and the potatoes and bring the pot to a boil.
3. Reduce the heat to a simmer and add the barley and lentils.
4. Simmer gently for 45 minutes, adding water if needed until the barley is plump and soft.
5. Serve hot.

Nutritional values per serving:

Calories 164, Fats 4 g, Carbohydrates 19 g, Proteins 5 g

Chickpea Noodle Soup

Prep time 8 minutes/ Cook time 5 minutes/ Serves 3

Ingredients:

- 1 tablespoon olive
- 1 clove garlic, minced
- 1 onion, diced
- 6 stalks celery, diced
- 4 carrots, peeled and diced
- 4 cups vegetable stock
- 4 cups water
- 2 heaping tablespoons white miso paste
- 4 ounces whole-wheat pasta
- 1 15-ounce can chickpeas, rinsed and drained
- salt and pepper to taste
- 2 handfuls baby spinach

Directions:

1. Place the oil in a large pot over medium high heat.
2. Sauté the garlic for one to two minutes, then add the onion and sauté for another couple minutes, until softened.
3. Add the celery and carrot and sauté for another two to three minutes.
4. Add the vegetable stock and water and bring the pot to a boil.

5. Pour in the pasta; as soon as it is cooked al dente, add the miso paste and chickpeas and turn down the heat to a simmer.
6. Season with salt and pepper to taste, simmering until everything is heated through.
7. If you are freezing your soup, stop here and let the soup cool before putting into freezer containers. However, if you plan to serve the soup immediately, toss in the spinach, turn off the heat and let the pot set there just long enough to wilt the spinach.
8. Serve the soup hot.

Nutritional values per serving:

Calories 120, Fats 3 g, Carbohydrates 5 g, Proteins 5 g

Creamy Carrot and White Bean Soup

Prep time 6 minutes/ Cook time 35 minutes/ Serves 5

Ingredients:

- 2 pounds carrots, peeled and chopped
- 2 tablespoons maple syrup
- 1 14-ounce can coconut milk
- 1½ cups vegetable stock
- 1 14-ounce can white beans
- 1 pinch turmeric
- 1 pinch curry powder
- 1 pinch salt
- 1 pinch pepper

Directions:

1. Preheat the oven to 350 degrees, Fahrenheit and line a rimmed baking sheet with parchment paper.
2. Place the chopped carrots in a bowl and pour in the maple syrup. Toss and make sure each carrot piece is coated with the syrup.
3. Spread the carrots on the baking sheet, making sure they don't overlap. Bake for 35 minutes.
4. Remove the carrots from the oven and cool for at least 15 minutes.
5. Scrape the carrots into a blender or food processor; add the coconut milk and vegetable stock and blend until smooth.

6. Add the beans, turmeric, curry, salt and pepper; blend until smooth and creamy.
7. Pour back into the pot and heat through before serving.

Nutritional values per serving:

Calories 130, Fats 5 g, Carbohydrates 19 g, Proteins 6 g

Creamy Leek and Potato Soup

Prep time 5 minutes/ Cook time 20 minutes/ Serves 3

Ingredients:

- 3 large leeks, cleaned and chopped in pieces
- 1 tablespoon vegan butter
- 1½ tablespoons olive oil
- 1 pinch sea salt
- 1 small onion, diced
- 3 medium potatoes, peeled and chopped
- 3 cloves garlic, minced
- ½ teaspoon dried rosemary
- 1½ teaspoons dried thyme
- ½ teaspoon ground coriander
- 5 cups vegetable stock
- 1 teaspoon more sea salt
- ¼ teaspoon pepper
- 2 bay leaves
- 1 cup coconut milk
- 1 green onion, chopped

Directions:

1. Prepare the leeks and drain them well
2. Put the butter and oil in a large pot over medium heat and add a pinch of salt.

3. When the butter is melted, add the leeks and onion and sauté for five to six minutes, until soft.
4. Add the potatoes, garlic, rosemary, thyme and coriander and sauté for about three minutes.
5. Pour in the vegetable broth, salt, pepper and bay leaves and bring to a boil.
6. Immediately turn the heat down to a simmer and let it cook for 15 minutes.
7. Remove the bay leaves and pour in the coconut milk. Taste and season with salt and pepper.
8. Use an immersion blender (or process in batches in a blender) and blend until smooth and creamy.
9. Pour back into the pot if it was removed; heat through until hot.
10. Ladle into bowls and top with chopped green onion and a little more pepper.

Nutritional values per serving:

Calories 340, Fats 6 g, Carbohydrates 29 g, Proteins 9 g

Green Cream of Broccoli Soup

Prep time 10 minutes/ Cook time 25 minutes/ Serves 4

Ingredients:

- 6 cups fresh broccoli florets
- 1 teaspoon olive
- 1 clove garlic, chopped
- 1 teaspoon tamari sauce
- 2 cups cold coconut milk
- 1 teaspoon dry Italian seasoning
- ¼ teaspoon sea salt
- ¼ teaspoon ground pepper
- 1 dash of cayenne pepper

Directions:

1. Cut up the broccoli into florets and place in a steamer basket over a pan of boiling water. Steam the florets for seven to eight minutes, until they are tender crisp.
2. Place oil in a large soup pot over medium heat and let it heat up. Add the garlic and sauté for about two minutes.
3. Add the tamari sauce and coconut milk, stir and add the steamed broccoli.
4. Add the Italian seasoning, salt and the black and cayenne pepper; turn off the heat while you use an immersion blender to process the mixture until it's smooth and creamy.

5. If the soup is too thick for your liking, add more coconut milk, two tablespoons at a time, until you get to the proper consistency.
6. Turn the burner back on over medium heat and simmer for 10 to 15 minutes.

Nutritional values per serving:

Calories 139, Fats 4 g, Carbohydrates 39 g, Proteins 8 g

Chilled Sweet Corn Soup

Prep time 10 minutes/ Cook time 0 minutes/ Serves 8

Ingredients:

- 12 fresh ears corn, shucked
- 1 teaspoon ground cinnamon
- 1 ½ cups sliced watermelon
- ½ cup fresh basil leaves
- 2 cups plain almond milk
- 8 tablespoons maple syrup
- ½ pint blackberries

Directions:

1. Remove the corn from the cobs. Add corn, cinnamon and milk into a blender and blend until smooth.
2. Pass the mixture thorough a nut milk bag and strain the milk into a bowl. Throw off the solids.
3. Add maple syrup and stir.
4. Divide into bowls. Divide the watermelon and blackberries into the bowls. Garnish with basil and refrigerate until use.

Nutritional values per serving:

Calories 258, Fats 4 g, Carbohydrates 57 g, Proteins 8 g

Pea and Mint Soup

Prep time 10 minutes/ Cook time 0 minutes/ Serves 8

Ingredients:

- 2 tablespoons extra-virgin olive oil
- 2 medium onions, finely chopped
- 10 cups shelled fresh peas
- 8 cups vegetable stock
- 2 ounces vegan butter
- 2 cloves garlic, peeled, minced
- 2 cups mint leaves
- Salt to taste
- Pepper to taste
- Vegan Parmesan cheese

Directions:

1. Place a soup pot over medium heat. Add oil and butter. When it heats, add onion and sauté until translucent.
2. Stir in the garlic and cook for about 2-3 minutes.
3. Add 8 cups peas, mint and 6 cups stock. Cover and cook until soft.
4. Turn off the heat and transfer into a blender. Blend until smooth.
5. Pour into the pot. Add rest of the stock and peas. Add salt and pepper to taste.
6. Place pot over medium heat. Cook until peas are soft.

7. Add cheese if using. Simmer until cheese melts.
8. Add a few drops of olive oil and stir.
9. Cool completely.
10. Ladle into bowls and serve.

Nutritional values per serving:

Calories 349, Fats 13 g, Carbohydrates 43 g, Proteins 17 g

Tomato and Basil Soup

Prep time 10 minutes/ Cook time 20 minutes/ Serves 8

Ingredients:

- 4 pounds tomatoes, quartered
- 4 cups vegetable broth
- 4 tablespoons balsamic vinegar
- Freshly ground pepper to taste
- 2 bunches fresh basil, chopped
- 4 cloves garlic, peeled
- Salt to taste

Directions:

1. Add all the ingredients into a blender and blend until the preferred consistency.
2. Strain if desired and pour into a large saucepan. Place over low heat. Let it cook for 20 minutes.
3. Cool completely and serve in bowls.

Nutritional values per serving:

Calories 110, Fats 1 g, Carbohydrates 22 g, Protein 6 g

Mushroom Barley Soup

Prep time 5 minutes/ Cook time 4 minutes/ Serves 6

Ingredients:

- 2 cups sliced fresh mushrooms
- 2 tablespoons vegan butter
- 2/3 cup medium pearl barley
- 2 medium carrots, sliced
- Salt to taste
- Pepper to taste
- 4 cloves garlic, minced
- 4 cans vegetable broth
- 2 tablespoons soy sauce
- 1 teaspoon dill weed

Directions:

1. Place a soup pot over medium heat. Add vegan butter. When it melts, add mushroom and garlic and sauté for about 3-4 minutes.
2. Add barley, broth and soy sauce.
3. When it begins to boil, lower the heat and cover the pot partially. Simmer until tender.
4. If the barley is not cooked and there is not sufficient broth, add more broth and cook until barley is tender.
5. Add carrot, dill, salt and pepper. Cover and cook until carrots are tender.

Nutritional values per serving:

Calories 230, Fats 6 g, Carbohydrates 34 g, Protein 12 g

Miso Soup

Prep time 10 minutes/ Cook time 8 minutes/ Serves 4

Ingredients:

- 4 cups water
- 1 cup chopped green onion
- 2 sheets dried nori, chopped
- 1 cup chopped green chard
- ½ cup cubed tofu
- 7-8 tablespoons white miso paste
- Salt to taste

Directions:

1. Add water into a saucepan. Place saucepan over high heat. When it begins to boil, add nori and cover with lid. Cook for 2-3 minutes.
2. Add green onion, green chard and tofu and cook for about 5 minutes. Turn off the heat.
3. Whisk together in a bowl, miso and hot water.
4. Pour into the hot soup. Stir and taste the soup. Add more salt or miso if desired.
5. Cool slightly.
6. Ladle into soup bowls and serve

Nutritional values per serving:

Calories 88, Fats 2 g, Carbohydrates 9 g, Proteins 7 g

Wonder Soup

Prep time 4 minutes/ Cook time 5 minutes/ Serves 6

Ingredients:

- 3 onions, chopped
- 2 medium tomatoes, chopped
- 1 medium bunch celery, trimmed, chopped
- 1 large green bell pepper, deseeded, chopped
- 1 medium cabbage, chopped into bite size pieces
- 1 medium carrot, chopped
- 1 cup sliced mushrooms
- Fresh or dried herbs of your choice
- Seasoning of your choice to taste
- Salt to taste
- 3 cups water

Directions:

1. Place a soup pot over medium heat.
2. Add all the ingredients and stir. Bring to a boil.
3. Lower the heat and simmer for 5 minutes until the vegetables are tender.
4. Ladle into soup bowls and serve.

Nutritional values per serving:

Calories 71, Fats 3.26 g, Carbohydrates 7.69 g, Proteins 3.92 g

Tortilla Soup

Prep time 5 minutes/ Cook time 20 minutes/ Serves 3

Ingredients:

- ½ cup salsa
- ½ teaspoon chili powder
- ½ can chickpeas, drained, rinsed
- 1 small onion, chopped
- 2 cups vegetable stock
- ½ teaspoon ground cumin
- Salt to taste
- ½ can corn, drained, rinsed
- 2 cloves garlic, minced
- Lime juice to taste
- Avocado slices
- Tortilla chips
- Chopped cilantro

Directions:

1. Add all the ingredients into a soup pot. Place the pot over medium heat.
2. Cover and simmer for 20-30 minutes.
3. Add lime juice and stir.
4. Ladle into soup bowls and serve with suggested toppings.

Nutritional values per serving:

Calories 237, Fats 4 g, Carbohydrates 39 g, Proteins 13 g

Greek Meatball Soup

Prep time 10 minutes/ Cook time 30 minutes/ Serves 4

Ingredients:

- ¾ cup dry brown lentils, rinsed
- ½ small onion, chopped
- 2 ½ cups vegetable broth
- Juice of a large lemon
- 2 tablespoons breadcrumbs
- Salt to taste
- Pepper to taste
- 7 tablespoons long grain brown rice
- ¼ cup flour
- ½ tablespoon cornstarch mixed with 2 tablespoons water
- 2 tablespoons parsley, chopped
- 1 tablespoon olive oil
- 1 tablespoon ground flaxseeds
- 2 cups water

Directions:

1. Add 2 cups broth and lentils into a saucepan and place over medium-high heat.
2. When it begins to boil, reduce the heat and simmer until lentils are cooked. Strain lentils and retain cooked water.

3. Place another small saucepan with 6 tablespoons rice and remaining broth and cook until rice is soft. Add half the rice into a blender.
4. Add the retained liquid back to the saucepan. Also add water and place over medium heat.
5. Meanwhile, add lentils into the blender and pulse until coarsely mashed.
6. Transfer into a bowl. Add remaining cooked rice, parsley, oil, breadcrumbs and flaxseeds and mix until well combined.
7. Divide the mixture 12 equal portions and shape into balls.
8. Add remaining tablespoon of uncooked rice to the simmering broth and lower the lentil balls into it.
9. Reduce heat and simmer for about 30 minutes.
10. Add cornstarch mixture to the simmering broth and stir gently. Add lemon juice, salt and pepper.
11. Ladle into soup bowls.

Nutritional values per serving:

Calories 461.8, Fats 5.75 g, Carbohydrates 51.6 g, Proteins 20 g

Creamy Curried Cauliflower Soup

Prep time 10 minutes/ Cook time 10 minutes/ Serves 3

Ingredients:

- 1 tablespoon extra-virgin olive oil + extra to serve
- 1 medium head cauliflower trimmed, chopped into florets
- 1 small white onion, thinly sliced
- 1 large clove garlic, peeled, minced
- 2 ¼ cups vegetable broth or water
- 1/3 cup fresh coconut milk
- ¾ teaspoon ground cumin
- ¼ teaspoon ground coriander
- ¼ teaspoon turmeric powder
- ½ teaspoon curry powder
- Salt to taste
- Freshly ground pepper to taste
- 2 tablespoons chopped, roasted cashew nuts
- 2 tablespoons chopped fresh Italian parsley
- ½ teaspoon red chili flakes to garnish

Directions:

1. Place a soup pot over medium heat. Add oil. When oil is heated, add onions and a large pinch of salt and sauté for 10 minutes until soft. Add garlic and sauté until aromatic.
2. Stir in the cauliflower, broth, coriander, curry powder, cumin, turmeric and salt. Mix well.

3. When it begins to boil, lower the heat and cover with a lid. Simmer until tender. Turn off the heat and cool for a while.
4. Transfer into a blender and blend until smooth. Pour the soup back into the pot.
5. Place the pot back over medium heat. Add coconut milk, and pepper and stir. Taste and adjust the seasoning if necessary.
6. Ladle into soup bowls. Sprinkle parsley, red pepper flakes and cashew nuts top
7. Drizzle some olive oil on top and serve immediately.

Nutritional values per serving:

Calories 177, Fats 13.2 g, Carbohydrates 14.2 g, Proteins 4.5 g

Lemongrass Lime Mushroom Soup

Prep time 6 minutes/ Cook time 21 minutes/ Serves 6

Ingredients:

- 1 tablespoon olive oil
- 1 tablespoon sesame oil
- 2 cloves garlic, minced
- ½ red onion, finely chopped
- 1 celery stalk, finely chopped
- 1 tablespoon fresh ginger, peeled and chopped
- 1 cup shitake mushrooms, thinly sliced
- 2 14-ounce cans coconut milk
- 1½ cups vegetable stock
- 1 small red chili pepper, seeded and minced
- 1 stalk fresh lemongrass, whole and pounded
- 1 to two tablespoons of lemongrass, minced
- Sea salt and ground pepper to taste
- 1 handful fresh basil leaves
- 1 lime, juiced
- ½ cup red bell pepper, julienned

Directions:

1. Place a soup pot over medium high heat and add the olive oil and sesame oil.
2. Sauté the garlic for one or two minutes, then add the onion, celery, ginger and mushrooms. Sauté for six minutes.

3. Add the coconut milk, vegetable broth, chili pepper, lemongrass stalk and minced lemongrass.
4. Season with salt and pepper.
5. Bring to a simmer and let it cook for around 15 minutes; you want everything to be piping hot.
6. Stir in the basil leaves and turn the heat off.
7. Squeeze in the lime juice, stir the pot and serve with a fresh basil leaf on top of each bowlful.

Nutritional values per serving:

Calories 200, Fats 4 g, Carbohydrates 39 g, Proteins 8 g

Chapter 8

Dinner Recipes

Chickpea Mushroom Pita Burgers

Prep time 10 minutes/ Cook time 30 minutes/ Serves 6

Ingredients:

Burgers:

- 6 pita breads
- 1 ½ cups cooked basmati rice
- 1 14-ounce can chickpeas
- 2 flax eggs
- 1 onion, chopped
- 4 cloves garlic, chopped
- 8 ounces mushrooms, chopped
- 2 tbsp soy sauce
- 1 ¼ cup chickpea flour

Spices:

- 1 tbsp coconut sugar
- ¼ cup nutritional yeast
- ½ tsp smoked paprika powder
- ½ tsp black pepper powder
- ½ tsp cumin powder

- ½ tsp coriander powder
- ¼ tsp allspice powder

Sauce:

- 2 tbsp vegan mayonnaise
- 1 tsp mustard
- 1 tsp gochujang
- Pinch of coconut sugar

Directions:

1. Cook the rice and sauté onion and garlic. Add mushrooms and salt until tender.
2. Drain chickpeas and add everything apart from chickpea flour to a food processor. Pulse until combined but not mushy.
3. Add this mixture to a bowl and add chickpea flour until everything is combined.
4. Form into patties.
5. Pan-fry the patties or bake them in an oven. Once done, assemble into the pita.
6. For the sauce, whisk everything together. Serve with the patties.

Nutritional values per serving: Calories 200, Fats 4 g, Carbohydrates 39 g, Proteins 8 g

Indian Mashed Potatoes

Prep time 10 minutes/ Cook time 30 minutes/ Serves 2

Ingredients:

- 2 pounds red potatoes
- 1 13-ounce can coconut milk
- 1/3 cup tomato sauce
- 2 tbsp olive oil
- 1 slice onion, chopped
- 1 tsp cumin seeds
- 1 tsp mustard seeds
- 1 tbsp coriander powder
- 1 tsp fenugreek powder
- 1 tsp turmeric powder
- Salt to taste
- Frozen peas for garnish

Directions:

1. Peel, chop, boil, and drain potatoes.
2. Sauté onion with salt.
3. Add cumin, mustard seeds, coriander powder, and turmeric. Mix well and take off from the heat.
4. Mash potatoes and add the spiced oil to them. Add salt to taste.
5. In a small pot, add a can of coconut milk and 1/3 cup tomato sauce. Mix 1 tsp each of turmeric, fenugreek, and coriander powder. Add salt and pepper to taste.
6. Pour curry gravy on potatoes and serve topped with green peas.

Nutritional values per serving: Calories 200, Fats 4 g, Carbohydrates 39 g, Proteins 8 g

Chickpeas and Spinach Andalusian Style

Prep time 10 minutes/ Cook time 15 minutes/ Serves 4

Ingredients:

- 1 ¾ cup fresh spinach
- 14-ounce can chickpeas
- 1 tbsp cumin seeds
- 1 tbsp smoked paprika
- Pinch fresh cayenne pepper
- 2 slices bread
- 3 cloves garlic, thinly sliced
- 1 tbsp Sherry vinegar
- 1 tbsp salt
- 1 tbsp ground black pepper
- 6 tbsp extra virgin olive oil

Directions:

1. Wash spinach and cook in boiling water for 3 minutes. Drain and set aside.
2. In a hot pan, heat olive oil and fry garlic until brown and crunchy. Set aside.
3. Using a mortar and pestle, grind together cumin seeds, salt, pepper, cayenne, bread, and garlic.
4. Add Sherry vinegar to the paste and a bit of water from the canned chickpeas.

5. Using the same saucepan, saute spinach before adding the rest of previous ingredients.
6. Stir until cooked.

Nutritional values per serving: Calories 200, Fats 4 g, Carbohydrates 39 g, Proteins 8 g

Zucchini Gratin

Prep time 10 minutes/ Cook time 20 minutes/ Serves 3

Ingredients:

Gratin:

- 6 medium zucchinis, thinly sliced
- 1 cup water
- ¾ cup raw cashews
- 2 tbsp apple cider vinegar
- 2 tbsp nutritional yeast
- 1 tsp garlic powder
- ½ tsp onion powder
- ¼ tsp black pepper
- Salt as needed

Toppings:

- 1 tbsp sesame seeds
- 1 tsp thyme

Directions:

1. Preheat oven to 400F.
2. Blend all ingredients, except zucchini and the toppings, until smooth to form a batter.
3. In a bowl, coat the zucchini slices in the batter.
4. Arrange the zucchinis in a baking pan or cast-iron skillet. Pour remaining batter over the zucchinis.
5. Bake for 20 minutes in the oven.
6. Add toppings and serve.

Nutritional values per serving: Calories 200, Fats 4 g, Carbohydrates 39 g, Proteins 8 g

Carrot Cashew Pate

Prep time 10 minutes/ Cook time 0 minutes/ Serves 4

Ingredients:

- 2 cups carrots, chopped into large pieces
- 1 cup cashews, soaked in water for an hour
- ¼ cup tahini
- ¼ cup lemon juice
- 1 tbsp peeled and grated ginger
- ½ cilantro, stems and leaves
- ½ tsp salt
- Bread or toast

Directions:

1. Place carrots in a food processor and blend until there are no big chunks.
2. Drain cashews and add into the processor with tahini, lemon juice, ginger, cilantro, and salt.
3. Process until completely smooth. Add salt to taste.
4. Serve on top of bread or toast.

Nutritional values per serving: Calories 200, Fats 4 g, Carbohydrates 39 g, Proteins 8 g

Cauliflower Steak with Sweet-pea Puree

Prep time 10 minutes/ Cook time 30 minutes/ Serves 2

Ingredients:

Cauliflower:

- 2 heads of cauliflower
- 1 tsp olive oil
- Paprika
- Coriander
- Black pepper

Sweet-pea puree:

- 1 10-ounce bag frozen green peas
- 1 small onion, chopped
- 2 tbsp fresh parsley
- ¼ cup unsweetened soy milk

Directions:

1. Preheat oven to 425F.
2. Remove bottom core of cauliflower. Stand it on its base, starting in the middle, slice in half. Then slice steaks about ¾ inches thick.
3. Place steaks on baking pan.
4. Lightly coat the front and back of each steak with olive oil.
5. Sprinkle with coriander, paprika, and pepper.
6. Bake for 30 minutes, flipping once.

7. Meanwhile, steam the chopped onion and peas until soft.
8. Place these vegetables in a blender with milk and parsley and blend until smooth.

Nutritional values per serving: Calories 200, Fats 4 g, Carbohydrates 39 g, Proteins 8 g

Taco Elbow Pasta

Prep time 10 minutes/ Cook time 0 minutes/ Serves 2

Ingredients:

- 1 ½ cups dry elbow pasta
- ½ can (from 15 ounces can) black beans, drained, rinsed
- 2 tomatoes, diced
- Avocado slices to serve (optional)
- 1 ½ cups vegetable stock
- 1 bell pepper, diced
- 1 teaspoon taco seasoning or to taste
- Water, as required

Directions:

1. Add all the ingredients into a pot. Place the pot over medium heat. Add water only if required. Cook until pasta is al dente.
2. Divide into bowls. Place avocado slices on top if using and serve.

Nutritional values per serving: Calories 200, Fats 4 g, Carbohydrates 39 g, Proteins 8 g

Vegan Lasagna

Prep time 10 minutes/ Cook time 60 minutes/ Serves 4

Ingredients:

For sauce:

- 1 tablespoon vegetable oil
- 1 ½ tablespoons minced garlic
- ¾ cup chopped onions
- 2 cans (14.5 ounces each) stewed tomatoes
- ¼ cup fresh basil
- ¼ cup fresh parsley
- Pepper to taste
- Salt to taste
- 3 tablespoons tomato paste

For lasagna:

- 8 ounces lasagna sheets, cooked according to the instructions on the package
- 1 tablespoon minced garlic
- 1-pound firm tofu, crumbled
- 1 ½ packages (10 ounces each) frozen spinach, thawed, squeezed of excess moisture
- Freshly ground pepper to taste
- Salt to taste
- 2 tablespoons chopped parsley

- 2 tablespoon chopped fresh basil
- ½ teaspoon Italian seasoning

Directions:

1. Place a skillet over medium heat. Add oil. When the oil is heated, add onions and sauté until translucent. Stir in the garlic and cook for another 3-4 minutes.
2. Add rest of the ingredients for sauce and stir. Lower the heat and cover with a lid. Cook for about 45 minutes. Stir occasionally. Turn off the heat.
3. For lasagna: To the crumbled tofu, add garlic, salt, pepper and fresh herbs. Mash well.
4. To assemble: Take a square or rectangular baking dish of about 8 inches. Spread about ½ cup sauce on the bottom of the dish.
5. Place a layer of lasagna noodles. Spread 1/3 the tofu mixture over it.
6. Your next layer should be of spinach.
7. Spread 10-12 tablespoons of the sauce.
8. Repeat step 5 and 7 twice. Your topmost layer will be of sauce.
9. Cover the dish with foil.
10. Bake in a preheated oven at 400° F for 25-30 minutes.

Nutritional values per serving: Calories 511, Fat 15.8 g, Carbohydrate 69.9 g, Protein 32.5 g

Creamy Cashew Alfredo

Prep time 8 minutes/ Cook time 20 minutes/ Serves 3

Ingredients:

For vegan Alfredo:

- ½ cup + 2 tablespoons raw cashews, soaked in hot water for 20 minutes, drained
- 2 tablespoons nutritional yeast
- Salt to taste
- ½ cup plain almond or rice milk or more if needed
- 1 ½ teaspoons arrowroot starch
- 1 clove garlic, crushed
- 1 tablespoon vegan Parmesan cheese

To assemble:

- 5 ounces fettuccini pasta, cooked
- Vegan Parmesan cheese, grated
- Roasted tomatoes to serve

Directions:

1. To make vegan Alfredo sauce: Add cashew, arrowroot, garlic, nutritional yeast, salt, nondairy milk and Parmesan into a blender and blend until smooth.
2. Taste and adjust garlic, nutritional yeast or vegan Parmesan and salt if required.

3. Pour into a saucepan. Place the saucepan over medium heat. Stir constantly until thick.
4. Add pasta and stir. Heat thoroughly.
5. Garnish with vegan Parmesan cheese and serve.
6. Serve with roasted tomatoes.

Nutritional values per: Calories 166, Fat 12.7 g, Carbohydrate 10.8 g, Protein 4.8 g

Zucchini Pasta

Prep time 10 minutes/ Cook time 3 minutes/ Serves 2

Ingredients:

- 1-pound large zucchinis, trimmed
- 1 medium onion, chopped
- ½ pint cherry tomatoes, halved
- 2 tablespoons extra virgin olive oil
- Zest of a lemon, grated
- ¼ cup basil leaves, finely sliced
- Freshly cracked pepper to taste
- Salt to taste
- 2 cloves garlic, minced
- Juice of a lemon
- ½ cup grated vegan Parmesan cheese
- Crushed red pepper to taste

Directions:

1. Make noodles of the zucchini using a spiralizer or a julienne peeler.
2. Place a skillet. Add oil. When the oil is heated, add garlic and onion and sauté until translucent.
3. Add zucchini and tomatoes and mix well. Cook for 2-3 minutes.
4. Add Parmesan, red pepper and basil.
5. Stir and serve.

Nutritional values per serving:

Calories 181, Fat 13.3 g, Carbohydrate 15.8 g, Protein 4.3 g

Spicy Peanut Soba Noodles

Prep time 7 minutes/ Cook time 17 minutes/ Serves 3

Ingredients:

- 5 ounces uncooked soba noodles
- ½ tablespoon low sodium soy sauce
- 1 clove garlic, minced
- 4 teaspoons water
- 1 small head broccoli, cut into florets
- ½ cup carrot
- ¼ cup finely chopped scallions
- 3 tablespoons peanut butter
- 1 tablespoon honey
- 1 teaspoon crushed red pepper flakes
- 2 teaspoons vegetable oil
- 4 ounces button mushrooms, discard stems
- 3 tablespoons peanuts, dry roasted, unsalted

Directions:

1. Cook soba noodles following the directions on the package.
2. Add peanut butter, honey, water, soy sauce, garlic and red pepper flakes. Whisk until well combined.
3. Place a skillet over medium heat. Add oil. When the oil is heated, add broccoli and sauté for a few minutes until crisp as well as tender.

4. Add mushrooms and sauté until the mushrooms are tender. Turn off the heat.
5. Add the sauce mixture and carrots and mix well.
6. Crush the peanuts by rolling with a rolling pin.
7. Divide the noodles into bowls. Pour sauce mixture over it. Sprinkle scallions and peanuts on top and serve.

Nutritional values per serving: Calories 280, Fat 11.3 g, Carbohydrates 39.2 g, Protein 11 g

Barbeque Bean Tacos with Tropical Salsa

Prep time 9 minutes/ Cook time 20 minutes/ Serves 3

Ingredients:

- 2 15-ounce cans pinto beans
- 1 tablespoon maple syrup
- 2 tablespoons prepared Dijon mustard
- ¾ cup ketchup
- ½ teaspoon chili powder
- ½ teaspoon garlic powder
- ¾ teaspoon sea salt, divided
- 1 20-ounce can pineapple chunks, packed in juice
- ¼ cup cilantro, finely chopped
- ¼ cup red onion, minced
- 3 radishes, stemmed and thinly sliced
- 1 small green cabbage, cored and thinly sliced
- 1 lime, cut into wedges
- 4 corn tortillas

Directions:

1. Drain and rinse the beans and pour into a heavy skillet.
2. Add the maple syrup, mustard, ketchup, chili powder, garlic powder and a half teaspoon of salt. Heat on low, stirring frequently, until the mixture heats through and thickens.
3. Meanwhile, drain and chop the pineapple chunks and put them in a bowl.

4. Add the cilantro, onion and the remaining salt and stir together.
5. Take a tortilla and place a fourth of the bean mixture on the side. Sprinkle with the radish and cabbage mixture and top with the pineapple mixture. Garnish the tops with more cilantro. Serve with lime wedges.

Nutritional values per serving: Calories 224, Fats 5g, Carbohydrates 29 g, Proteins 12 g

Burgundy Mushroom Sauce Over Polenta

Prep time 7 minutes/ Cook time 15 minutes/ Serves 4

Ingredients:

- 1 tablespoon olive oil
- 1 medium red onion, chopped
- 4 cloves garlic, minced
- 2 large carrots, peeled, cut in half and thinly sliced
- 24 ounces Cremini mushrooms, sliced
- 1 teaspoon dry mustard
- ½ teaspoon dried rosemary
- ½ teaspoon dried thyme
- ½ teaspoon sea salt
- ½ teaspoon ground black pepper
- 1½ cups red wine
- 1 15-ounce can diced tomatoes
- 2 tablespoon Worcestershire sauce
- 4 green onions, chopped
- 1 cup unsweetened non-dairy milk
- ¼ cup parsley, chopped

Directions:

1. In a large pot over medium heat, heat the olive oil and the onion. Sauté for two to three minutes.

2. Add the garlic, carrots, dry mustard, rosemary, thyme, salt and pepper and sauté until the mushrooms turn golden and lose most of their liquid.
3. Deglaze with the wine; scrape the brown bits up from the bottom of the pan.
4. Add the tomatoes, Worcestershire sauce and green onions. Cook to reduce the liquid by half.
5. Make some polenta, rice, or quinoa and set it aside until ready to serve.
6. If you're using polenta, stir in enough of the non-dairy milk or vegetable broth until it becomes the consistency of mashed potatoes.
7. To serve, spoon the mushroom sauce over the polenta and sprinkle with the parsley.

Nutritional values per serving:

Calories 243, Fats 6 g, Carbohydrates 23 g, Proteins 10 g

Carrot Brown Rice Casserole With Spinach

Prep time 7 minutes/ Cook time 55 minutes/ Serves 4

Ingredients:

- 1 bunch fresh spinach leaves, chopped
- 2 tablespoons vegetable stock
- 3 cups shredded carrots
- 1 large onion, chopped
- 1 teaspoon sea salt
- ½ teaspoon dry thyme
- 1½ teaspoons garlic powder
- ¼ cup smooth peanut butter
- 3 cups water or vegetable stock
- 3 cups cooked brown rice
- 1 tablespoon soy sauce
- ¾ cup whole-grain crumbs

Directions:

1. Coat the inside of a two-quart casserole with nonstick spray and preheat the oven to 350 degrees, Fahrenheit.
2. Spread the spinach on the bottom of the casserole dish.
3. Heat a large pot over medium high heat and add the two tablespoons of vegetable broth. This will keep everything from sticking to the pan.
4. Add the onions and carrots and sauté for five minutes.
5. Add the salt, thyme and garlic powder and stir in.

6. Add the peanut butter and water or vegetable stock and whisk until smooth.
7. Stir in the soy sauce along with the breadcrumbs and stir well.
8. Pour this on top of the spinach and cover with a lid or foil.
9. Bake for 45 minutes and take out of the oven. Let cool for 10 minutes, remove the cover and serve.

Nutritional values per serving: Calories 241, Fats 11 g, Carbohydrates 20 g, Proteins 16g

Cashew Topped Vegetable Stuffed Peppers

Prep time 10 minutes/ Cook time 60 minutes/ Serves 5

Ingredients:

- 1 tablespoon olive oil
- 2 cloves garlic, chopped
- 1 medium onion, chopped
- 8 ounces mushrooms, sliced
- 2 to three large Swiss chard leaves, coarsely chopped
- 1 15-ounce can kidney beans, rinsed and drained
- 8 sun-dried tomatoes, soaked
- 1 to 2 cups tomato sauce
- 1½ cups cooked brown rice or quinoa
- 3 large red peppers, cut into half lengthwise
- 1/3 cup raw cashews, finely chopped

Directions:

1. Preheat the oven to 375 degrees, Fahrenheit.
2. Place the olive oil in a heated skillet and add the garlic, sautéing for two minutes.
3. Add the onions and mushrooms and sauté until the onion is soft.
4. Add the chard and beans and cook until the chard wilts.
5. Add the drained and chopped sun-dried tomatoes, tomato sauce and cooked rice or quinoa. Stir to combine everything.
6. Fill the pepper cups with the mixture and place in a baking dish that has been sprayed with nonstick spray. Cover with foil.

7. Bake for 40 minutes, remove from the oven and sprinkle cashews over the top. Bake for another 10 minutes.
8. Cool for 10 minutes before serving.

Nutritional values per serving: Calories 321, Fats 7 g, Carbohydrates 22 g, Proteins 15g

Coconut Curry With Cauliflower and Tomato

Prep time 10 minutes/ Cook time 30 minutes/ Serves 6

Ingredients:

- Cooked brown rice for serving
- 2 tablespoons olive oil
- 1 onion, chopped
- 1 pound (about 4 cups) sweet potato, unpeeled but chopped
- 1 head cauliflower (about 4 cups), chopped
- 1 teaspoon kosher salt, divided
- 1 tablespoon garam masala
- 1 teaspoon cumin
- ¼ teaspoon cayenne pepper
- 2 tablespoons curry powder
- 1 23-ounce jar diced San Marzano plum tomatoes
- 1 15-ounce can full-fat coconut milk
- 1 15-ounce can chickpeas, rinsed and drained
- 4 cups fresh spinach leaves
- Cilantro for garnish

Directions:

1. Heat the oil in a large pot over medium heat.
2. Sauté the onions for about three minutes, then add the sweet potato and sauté for another 3 minutes.
3. Add the cauliflower and a half teaspoon of the salt; sauté for five minutes.

4. Add the garam marsala, cumin, cayenne pepper and curry powder; stir to mix thoroughly.
5. Pour in the plum tomatoes, including their juice and the coconut milk; bring to a boil.
6. Reduce the heat and simmer, covered, for about 10 minutes. The cauliflower should be soft.
7. Add the chickpeas and spinach leaves, along with the rest of the salt; stir until the spinach wilts and the chickpeas are heated through.
8. Serve over brown rice and garnish with cilantro.

Nutritional values per serving: Calories 315, Fats 9g, Carbohydrates 32 g, Proteins 11g

Greek Style Stuffed Sweet Potatoes

Prep time 10 minutes/ Cook time 30 minutes/ Serves 4

Ingredients:

- 4 sweet potatoes
- ½ red onion, chopped
- 1 cucumber, peeled and chopped
- 2 large tomatoes, chopped
- 1 small jar Kalamata olives, chopped
- 3 tablespoons fresh mint, chopped
- 1 lime, juiced
- 1 clove garlic, processed into a paste
- 2 tablespoons lemon juice
- 1/3 cup Tahini sauce
- ¼ teaspoon salt
- 2 to 6 tablespoons lukewarm water
- 1 15-ounce can chickpeas, drained and rinsed

Directions:

1. Preheat the oven to 375 degrees, Fahrenheit.
2. Cut the cleaned sweet potatoes in half lengthwise and place them, with cut side down, on a greased baking sheet. Bake for 20 to 30 minutes, until tender when poked with a fork. Remove from the oven to cool.
3. In a bowl, combine the onions, cucumber, tomatoes, olives, mint and lime juice. Mix well and set the bowl aside.

4. In another bowl, combine the garlic, lemon juice, Tahini sauce and salt. Start adding the water with two tablespoons and see if it becomes the right consistency. If it is thick and pasty, add more of the water up to six tablespoons. Set the mixture aside.
5. To assemble, place two potato halves on a plate right side up and mash with a fork lightly. Place the onion, cucumber tomato and olive mixture on top. Sprinkle with chickpeas and end up with the Tahini mixture on top and serve.

Nutritional values per serving: Calories 200, Fats 4 g, Carbohydrates 39 g, Proteins 8 g

Imitation Crab Cakes With Tofu

Prep time 8 minutes/ Cook time 20 minutes/ Serves 4

Ingredients:

- 2 tablespoons ground flaxseed
- 4 tablespoons water
- 1 block tofu
- ½ cup red bell pepper, diced
- ½ cup yellow bell pepper, diced
- ¾ cup red onion, diced
- 1½ cups celery diced
- ¼ cup flat leaf parsley, chopped
- 1 tablespoons capers, drained
- ½ teaspoon Worcestershire sauce
- ¼ teaspoon hot sauce
- 1½ teaspoons Old Bay seasoning
- ¼ cup vegetable stock
- salt and pepper to taste
- 1 tablespoon lemon juice
- ½ tablespoon lemon zest
- ½ cup dry wheat bread crumbs
- 2 tablespoons Dijon mustard
- Mango salsa, for accompaniment

Directions:

1. Combine the flaxseed and water and let it soak until ready to use.
2. Cut the tofu block in half lengthwise, pressing each half between paper towels and wrapping in newspaper to make it as dry as possible. Place something heavy on top and let it rest for 20 minutes.
3. Put the red and yellow bell pepper, the onion, celery, parsley, capers, Worcestershire sauce, hot sauce, Old Bay seasoning, vegetable stock, salt and pepper in a large pot over medium low heat. Cook for 15 minutes or until everything is soft. Cool to room temperature.
4. Place the tofu in a large bowl and mash it into small pieces
5. Add the lemon juice, lemon zest, breadcrumbs, mustard and the flaxseed, including the water. Mix well.
6. Add the vegetable mixture and mix well.
7. Cover the bowl and let it rest in the refrigerator for 30 minutes.
8. Preheat the oven to 375 degrees, Fahrenheit and cover a baking sheet with parchment paper.
9. Remove the mixture from the refrigerator and shape it into balls, place them on the parchment paper and press down to flatten.
10. Bake for five minutes on each side and serve with mango salsa.

Nutritional values per serving: Calories 278, Fats 8 g, Carbohydrates 26 g, Proteins 12g

Lentil and Mushroom Loaf (Fake Meatloaf)

Prep time 10 minutes/ Cook time 60 minutes/ Serves 8

Ingredients:

- 2 cloves garlic, finely chopped
- 1 small onion, chopped
- 3 cups mushrooms, finely chopped
- 1 cup green lentils, already cooked
- 1 cup red lentils, already cooked
- ½ cup old-fashioned rolled oats
- ¼ cup ground flaxseed
- 1 tablespoon Tamari or soy sauce
- 2 tablespoons dried thyme
- ½ teaspoon salt
- ¼ teaspoon pepper
- 2 tablespoons to ½ cup water

Directions:

1. Preheat the oven to 370 degrees, Fahrenheit.
2. Place the garlic, onion and mushrooms in a large mixing bowl.
3. Add the green and red lentils, oats, flaxseed, Tamari, thyme, salt and pepper; mix well with your hands. The mixture may be a little crumbly.
4. Add water, a little bit at a time and up to a half cup as needed until the mixture starts to stick together like a regular meatloaf.

Add two tablespoons first, then add by two-tablespoon increments until the loaf gains the proper texture.

5. Place a strip of parchment paper on the bottom of the pan that extends up both sides and out of the pan on the small sides. This creates a sling that you can grasp to pull out the loaf after it's cooked.
6. Pack the loaf mixture into the pan and bake for 50 to 60 minutes.
7. Remove from oven and cool for 15 minutes. Lift the loaf out of the pan and set it on a cutting board to slice Serve while warm.

Nutritional values per serving: Calories 324, Fats 12g, Carbohydrates 32 g, Proteins 11g

Meatless Chick Nuggets

Prep time 10 minutes/ Cook time 30 minutes/ Serves 8

Ingredients:

- 1 15.5-ounce can chickpeas, rinsed and drained
- ½ teaspoon garlic powder
- 1 teaspoon granulated onion
- 1 tablespoon nutritional yeast
- 1 tablespoon whole-wheat bread crumbs
- ½ cup panko bread crumbs

Directions:

1. Preheat the oven to 350 degrees, Fahrenheit and cover a rimmed baking pan with parchment paper.
2. Place the drained chickpeas in a food processor and pulse four to five times.
3. Add the garlic powder, granulated onion, nutritional yeast and the tablespoon of whole-wheat bread crumbs to the processor and process until you get a chunky, grainy mixture that sticks together.
4. Scoop out by teaspoonfuls and form balls.
5. Roll the balls in the panko crumbs and set on the baking sheet, flattening each ball so it looks more like a chicken nugget. Be sure to space them apart so they do not touch each other.

6. Bake for 20 minutes, remove from the oven and flip each nugget over with tongs. Return to the oven for 10 more minutes.
7. Cool for a few minutes and then serve with honey, barbecue sauce or Ranch dipping sauce.

Nutritional values per serving: Calories 365, Fats 8g, Carbohydrates 21g, Proteins 16g

Portobello Bolognese With Zucchini Noodles

Prep time 6 minutes/ Cook time 25 minutes/ Serves 4

Ingredients:

- 3 tablespoons olive oil, divided
- ½ cup onion, minced
- 3 cloves of garlic, minced
- ½ cup carrot, peeled and minced
- ½ cup celery, minced
- 6 portobello mushroom caps, stems removed and finely chopped
- ½ teaspoon Kosher salt
- ½ teaspoon ground pepper
- 1 tablespoon tomato paste
- 1 28-ounce can crushed plum tomatoes
- ¼ teaspoon red pepper flakes, crushed
- ½ cup fresh basil leaves, finely chopped
- 2 teaspoons dried oregano
- 4 medium zucchini

Directions:

1. Heat two tablespoons of the olive oil in a large skillet over medium high heat.
2. Add the onion, garlic, carrot and celery; sauté for about five minutes or until the onion turns translucent.

3. Add the mushrooms and sauté for another six to seven minutes, until the mushrooms shrink and lose their liquid. Stir constantly so they don't burn but turn a golden hue.
4. Stir in the tomato paste and cook, stirring frequently, for about two minutes.
5. Pour in the crushed tomatoes, red pepper flakes, basil and oregano. Reduce the heat to a simmer, cooking very low until the sauce thickens.
6. While the pot simmers, create the zucchini noodles and put them in cold water until they're all made. Drain the noodles and use tongs to place them in a skillet with a little water at the bottom. Toss and add some salt and pepper. They will only take a few minutes to soften and warm over medium heat.
7. Divide the noodles among four bowls and serve with the sauce on top; add a basil leaf on top as garnish.

Nutritional values per serving: Calories 352, Fats 5g, Carbohydrates 23g, Proteins 12g

Quesadilla With Black Beans and Sweet Potato

Prep time 10 minutes/ Cook time 30 minutes/ Serves 2

Ingredients:

- 1 medium-sized sweet potato, peeled and cut into cubes
- 3 teaspoons taco seasoning
- 4 whole-wheat tortillas
- ½ of a 15-ounce can of black beans, drained and rinsed
- Salsa for serving

Directions:

1. Bring a large pot of water to boil and drop in the sweet potato.
2. Boil for 10 to 20 minutes or until soft.
3. Drain the sweet potato and put in a bowl.
4. Add the taco seasoning and mash well.
5. To assemble the quesadilla, spread the sweet potato mixture on the tortilla.
6. Add the black beans and press them onto the potato mixture.
7. Cover with another tortilla.
8. Heat a nonstick skillet over medium high heat and lay the tortilla in it. Toast on both sides and serve immediately.

Nutritional values per serving: Calories 412, Fats 13g, Carbohydrates 27 g, Proteins 22g

Quinoa-stuffed Acorn Squash

Prep time 10 minutes/ Cook time 80 minutes/ Serves 4

Ingredients:

- ½ cup quinoa, cooked per package instructions
- 2 acorn squash
- 1/8 cup water
- 1 large onion, chopped
- 1/8 teaspoon ground cloves
- 1/8 teaspoon ground cardamom
- ½ teaspoon ground ginger
- 1 teaspoon ground cinnamon
- ½ cup raisins
- 1/3 cup walnuts or pecans, chopped
- ½ teaspoon sea salt
- ¼ teaspoon ground black pepper

Directions:

1. Preheat the oven to 350 degrees, Fahrenheit and pre-cook the quinoa. Set it aside until ready to use.
2. Poke the squash with a fork or knife to let the steam out (and to avoid a squash explosion). Place on a microwave safe dish and microwave on high for three to four minutes. This will soften the squash before you cut into it.
3. Let the squash cool for five minutes and then cut it in half. Carefully remove the seeds as they will still be hot. Place the

halves, cut side down, on a parchment-lined baking sheet. Bake for 30 to 40 minutes, until the squash is soft.

4. While squash is cooking, pour the water into a skillet over medium high heat and sauté the onion.
5. Reduce the heat to low and add the cloves, cardamom, ginger and cinnamon, stirring to mix. Turn off the heat and set the mixture aside until the squash is finished baking.
6. Once the squash is soft inside, remove it from the oven, but do not turn off the heat. As soon as it can be handled, carefully scoop the squash meat from the shell without damaging the skin. Mash the squash meat.
7. Add the squash meat to the onion spice mix in the skillet and turn the heat back on to medium high, stirring to mix.
8. Add the raisins and nuts and stir while heating through. Season with salt and pepper.
9. Turn off the heat and pack the shells with the mixture in the pan. Put the squash shells back on the baking sheet, cover everything with foil and bake for another 20 minutes before serving.

Nutritional values per serving: Calories 432, Fats 11 g, Carbohydrates 32 g, Proteins 16 g

Spicy Corn and Spinach Casserole

Prep time 12 minutes/ Cook time 80 minutes/ Serves 6

Ingredients:

- 1½ cups water
- ¾ cup unsweetened soy milk, divided
- 1¼ cups cornmeal
- 1 14-ounce block tofu, drained and rinsed
- 3 cloves garlic, minced
- 1 10-ounce package frozen corn, thawed, divided
- 2 4.5-ounce cans mild chilies, diced
- 1 10-ounce package frozen spinach, thawed, with the liquid squeezed out
- 1 teaspoon baking powder
- ½ teaspoon cayenne pepper
- ½ teaspoon cumin
- ½ teaspoon salt
- ½ teaspoon pepper
- Salsa as accompaniment

Directions:

1. Preheat the oven to 450 degrees, Fahrenheit.
2. Heat the water and a half cup of the soy milk in a medium saucepan, bringing it almost to a boil. Turn off the burner and slowly whisk in the cornmeal, letting It thicken. Scrape out into a bowl and set it aside until ready to use.

3. Wrap the tofu in a paper towel and press down to extract most of the liquid. This may require repeating several times, with fresh paper towels.
4. When the tofu is as dry as you can get it, place it in a food processor, along with the garlic, one cup of corn and the remaining soy milk. Process until smooth, then pour it into the bowl with the cornmeal, folding it in to combine thoroughly.
5. To the same bowl, add the rest of the corn, the chilies, spinach, baking powder, cayenne pepper, cumin, salt and pepper. The mixture will be thick but needs to be combined well. Use your muscles.
6. Pour the mixture into an oiled baking dish and bake for 60 to 70 minutes. The edges should be crispy and the middle should jiggle just a little bit.
7. Let the casserole stand for 20 minutes before serving with salsa.

Nutritional values per serving: Calories 432, Fats 9 g, Carbohydrates 24 g, Proteins 29g

Chapter 9

Dessert and Snacks Recipes

Mango & Papaya After-Chop

Prep time 25 minutes/ Cook time 0 minutes/ Serves 1

Ingredients:

- ¼ of papaya, chopped
- 1 mango, chopped
- 1 Tbsp coconut milk
- ½ tsp maple syrup
- 1 Tbsp peanuts, chopped

Directions:

1. Cut open the papaya. Scoop out the seeds, chop.
2. Peel the mango. Slice the fruit from the pit, chop.
3. Put the fruit in a bowl. Add remaining ingredients. Stir to coat.

Nutritional values per serving: Calories 100, Fats 1 g, Carbohydrates 25 g, Proteins 1 g

Sautéed Bosc Pears with Walnuts

Prep time 15 minutes/ Cook time 16 minutes/ Serves 6

Ingredients:

- 2 Tbsp salted butter
- ¼ tsp cinnamon
- ¼ tsp nutmeg, ground
- 6 Bosc pears, peeled, quartered
- 1 Tbsp lemon juice
- ½ cup walnuts, chopped, toasted

Directions:

1. Melt butter in a skillet, add spices and cook for 30 seconds.
2. Add pears and cook for 15 minutes. Stir in lemon juice.
3. Serve topped with walnuts.

Nutritional values per serving: Calories 220, Fats 10 g, Carbohydrates 31 g, Proteins 2 g

Brown Rice Pudding

Prep time 5 minutes/ Cook time 1 hour 30 minutes/ Serves 6

Ingredients:

- 2 cups brown rice, cooked
- 3 cups light coconut milk
- 3 eggs
- 1 cup brown sugar
- 1 tsp vanilla
- ½ tsp salt
- ½ tsp cinnamon
- ¼ tsp nutmeg

Directions:

1. Blend all ingredients well. Put mixture in a 2-quart casserole dish.
2. Bake at 300°F for 90 minutes.
3. Serve.

Nutritional values per serving: Calories 330, Fats 10 g, Carbohydrates 52 g, Proteins 5 g

Plant-based Taco Salad

Prep time 7 minutes/ Cook time 30 minutes/ Serves 3

Ingredients:

- 1 15-ounce can chickpeas, rinsed, drained and dried well in a paper towel
- 2 teaspoon cumin, divided
- 2 teaspoons chili powder, divided
- ½ teaspoon sea salt, divided
- ¼ teaspoon ground cinnamon
- 1 15-ounce can black beans, rinsed and drained
- ½ teaspoon garlic powder
- ½ teaspoon paprika
- ½ teaspoon cayenne
- ¼ cup water
- 1 head Romaine lettuce, chopped
- 1 red bell pepper, diced
- 1 tomato, chopped
- 1 cup frozen corn kernels, thawed, drained and patted dried
- 1 avocado, diced
- Creamy Ranch Dressing

Directions:

1. Preheat the oven to 400 degrees, Fahrenheit and prepare a lipped baking sheet by covering the surface with parchment paper.

2. In a bowl, sprinkle the drained chickpeas with one teaspoon of the cumin, one teaspoon of the chili powder, a quarter teaspoon of the sea salt and the cinnamon. Toss to coat.
3. Pour this mixture onto the prepared baking sheet, spreading the chickpeas in a single layer. Bake for 10 minutes. Shake the pan to turn over the chickpeas and bake for another 10 minutes. Remove from the oven and let cool.
4. Toss the black beans with the remaining garlic powder and salt, the paprika and the cayenne pepper; pour into a skillet over medium heat. Add the water and stir, cooking for five to six minutes, until warmed through. Set the pan aside.
5. In a large bowl, toss the lettuce, bell pepper, tomatoes, corn and avocado.
6. Place the lettuce in four separate bowls. Spoon the warm black bean mixture on top and sprinkle with the chickpeas.
7. Drizzle on top as much dressing as you please and stir it in.

Nutritional values per serving: Calories 322, Fats 7 g, Carbohydrates 30 g, Proteins 21 g

Raw Energy Squares

Prep time 30 minutes/ Cook time 0 minutes/ Serves 6

Ingredients:

- 2 cups Medjool dates, chopped and pitted
- 2 cups cashews
- ½ cup almonds
- ¾ cup powder, cocoa
- Sea salt, to taste
- 2 Tbsp vanilla extract
- 3 Tbsp cold water

Directions:

1. Blend first five ingredients in a food processor.
2. Add the vanilla and water, give a quick pulse.
3. Put the dough into a pan, making an even layer.
4. Cut into squares and serve.

Nutritional values per serving: Calories 330, Fats 10 g, Carbohydrates 52 g, Proteins 5 g

Spiced Pecans

Prep time 15 minutes/ Cook time 15 minutes/ Serves 12

Ingredients:

- 2 Tbsp brown sugar
- ½ tsp sweet paprika
- ½ tsp chili powder
- ½ cup butter, melted
- 4 cups pecans

Directions:

1. Preheat oven to 350°F.
2. Blend first five ingredients.
3. Pour in the butter and mix. Add the nuts and toss to coat.
4. Spread the seasoned nuts on a baking sheet. Roast for 15 minutes.

Nutritional values per serving: Calories 232, Fats 24 g, Carbohydrates 6 g, Proteins 2 g

Date Porcupines

Prep time 20 minutes/ Cook time 15 minutes/ Serves 18

Ingredients:

- 2 eggs
- 1 Tbsp extra-virgin olive oil
- 1 tsp vanilla
- 1 cup Medjool dates, pitted, chopped
- 1 cup walnuts, chopped
- ¾ cup flour
- 1 cup coconut, shredded
- ½ tsp salt

Directions:

1. Preheat oven to 350°F.
2. Beat the eggs, adding the oil and vanilla. Fold in the dates and walnuts. Add flour and salt to the mixture, mix well.
3. Form the mixture into small balls and roll in coconut. Bake for 15 minutes.
4. Serve cold.

Nutritional values per serving:

Calories 114, Fats 1 g, Carbohydrates 8 g, Proteins 1 g

Raspberry Chia Pudding Shots

Prep time 1 hour / Cook time 15 minutes/ Serves 2

Ingredients:

- ¼ cup chia seeds
- ½ cup raspberries
- ½ cup coconut milk
- ¼ cup almond milk
- 1 Tbsp cacao powder
- 1 Tbsp stevia

Directions:

1. Combine all ingredients except raspberries in a jar.
2. Let sit for 2-3 minutes and transfer to shot glasses.
3. Refrigerate 1 hour, or overnight to serve as breakfast.
4. Serve with fresh raspberries.

Nutritional values per serving: Calories 240, Fats 19 g, Carbohydrates 5 g, Proteins 5 g

Banana Muffins

Prep time 15 minutes/ Cook time 15 minutes/ Serves 18

Ingredients:

- 3 bananas
- 2 eggs
- 2 cups whole wheat pastry flour
- 1/3 cup sugar
- 1 tsp salt
- 1 tsp baking soda
- ½ cup walnuts, chopped

Directions:

1. Preheat oven to 350°F.
2. Grease and flour 10 cups of a muffin tin.
3. Mix bananas and eggs together. Add sifted dry ingredients.
4. Add nuts. Mix well.
5. Spoon into muffin tins. Bake for 20 minutes.

Nutritional values per serving: Calories 108, Fats 1 g, Carbohydrates 8 g, Proteins 1 g

Avocado-based Chocolate Mousse

Prep time 7 minutes/ Cook time 0 minutes/ Serves 3

Ingredients:

- 4 ripe avocados
- 1 cup agave syrup, divided
- 1 cup cacao, divided
- ¼ teaspoon salt
- ¼ teaspoon vanilla extract

Directions:

1. Prepare the avocados and place the meat in a food processor. Process until smooth.
2. Add half the agave syrup, half the cacao, the salt and the vanilla; process until smooth.
3. Taste to see if it needs more agave syrup or cacao and add anything that's lacking.
4. Refrigerate for at least two hours, or overnight, before serving.

Nutritional values per serving: Calories 354, Fats 6 g, Carbohydrates 11 g, Proteins 10 g

Banana Creamy Pie

Prep time 10 minutes/ Cook time 0 minutes/ Serves 4

Ingredients:

- 2 large pitted dates
- 1 pre-made pie crust, cooled
- 2 very ripe bananas, peeled and sliced, plus one a little less ripe for garnish
- 1 tablespoon coconut sugar
- 1 can coconut milk
- ½ teaspoon vanilla
- 1 pinch salt

Directions:

1. Soak the dates for about an hour, then drain and dry them.
2. Place the dates and banana slices in a food processor and pulse to break them up.
3. Add the coconut sugar, coconut milk, vanilla and salt and process until smooth and creamy.
4. Pour the filling into a cooled pie crust. It must be cool, or it will make the crust soggy.
5. Cover with plastic wrap and place the pie in the freezer for at least two hours.
6. Remove from the freezer and let it thaw a bit. Slice the remaining banana and place it on top. Serve while still partially frozen.

Nutritional values per serving:

Calories 131, Fats 3 g, Carbohydrates 15 g, Proteins 5g

Banana Mango Ice Cream

Prep time 30 minutes/ Cook time 0 minutes/ Serves 2

Ingredients:

- 1 banana, peeled and sliced
- 2 ripe mangos with the skin removed and the flesh cubed
- 3 tablespoons almond or cashew milk, chilled

Directions:

1. Lay out the banana and mango slices on a baking sheet lined with parchment paper and place them in the freezer.
2. Once they are frozen solid, remove the fruit and place it in the food processor.
3. Add the cold milk and process until smooth, about three to four minutes.
4. Taste and add sweetener as needed.
5. Serve immediately.

Nutritional values per serving: Calories 112, Fats 5 g, Carbohydrates 7 g, Proteins 8 g

Plant-Power Chopped Salad

Prep time 10 minutes/ Cook time 0 minutes/ Serves 3

Ingredients:

- 1 large head of Romaine lettuce, washed and chopped
- 2 cups baby arugula, chopped
- 1 medium zucchini, ends cut off and cut into slices
- 1 14-ounce can artichoke hearts, drained, dried and chopped
- 1 14-ounce can chickpeas, rinsed, drained and dried
- 2 medium carrots, peeled, quartered lengthwise and thinly sliced
- ¾ cup tomatoes, diced
- salt and pepper as desired
- 4 tablespoons shelled sunflower seeds

Directions:

1. Place the chopped lettuce in a large salad bowl; add the arugula and toss to mix.
2. Add the zucchini, artichoke hearts, chickpeas, carrots and tomatoes; toss to combine.
3. Add salt and pepper to your liking and sprinkle the top with sunflower seeds.
4. Serve with creamy ranch dressing

Nutritional values per serving: Calories 154, Fats 3 g, Carbohydrates 11 g, Proteins 3 g

Chapter 10

Plant Based Smoothies

Amazing Blueberry Smoothie

Prep time 5 minutes/ Serves 2

Ingredients:

- ½ avocado
- 1 cup, frozen blueberries
- 1 cup, raw spinach
- Pinch, sea salt
- 1 cup, soy
- 1 frozen banana

Directions:

1. Blend everything in a powerful blender until you have a smooth, creamy shake.
2. Enjoy your healthy shake and start your morning on a fresh note!

Nutritional value per serving:

Calories: 220, Fats 9 g, Carbohydrates 32 g, Proteins 5 g

Go-Green Smoothie

Prep time 5 minutes/ Serves 1

Ingredients:

- 2 tablespoons, natural cashew butter
- 1 ripe frozen banana
- 2/3 cup, unsweetened coconut
- 1 large handful, kale

Directions:

1. Put everything inside a powerful blender.
2. Blend until you have a smooth, creamy shake.
3. Enjoy your special green smoothie.

Nutritional value per serving:

Calories: 390, Fats 19 g, Carbohydrates 42 g, Proteins 15 g

Creamy Chocolate Shake

Prep time 10 minutes/ Serves 2

Ingredients:

- 2 frozen ripe bananas, chopped
- 1/3 cup frozen strawberries
- 2 tbsp cocoa powder
- 2 tbsp salted almond butter
- 2 cups unsweetened vanilla almond milk
- 1 dash Stevia or agave nectar
- 1/3 cup ice

Directions:

1. Add all ingredients in a blender and blend until smooth.
2. Take out and serve.

Nutritional value per serving:

Calories 312, Carbohydrates 48 g, Fats 14 g, Proteins 6.2 g

Hidden Kale Smoothie

Prep time 5 minutes/ Serves 2

Ingredients:

- 1 medium ripe banana, peeled and sliced
- ½ cup frozen mixed berries
- 1 tbsp hulled hemp seeds
- 2 cups frozen or fresh kale
- 2/3 cup 100% pomegranate juice
- 2¼ cups filtered water

Directions:

1. Add all ingredients in a blender and blend until smooth.
2. Take out and serve.

Nutritional value per serving:

Calories 178, Carbohydrates 37.8 g, Fats 1.8 g, Proteins 4.1 g

Blueberry Protein Shake

Prep time 5 minutes/ Serves 1

Ingredients:

- ½ cup cottage cheese
- 3 tbsp vanilla protein powder
- ½ cup frozen blueberries
- ½ tsp maple extract
- ¼ tsp vanilla extract
- 2 tsp flaxseed meal
- Sweetener, choice
- 10-15 ice cubes
- ¼ cup water

Directions:

1. Add all ingredients in a blender and blend until smooth.
2. Take out and serve.

Nutritional value per serving:

Calories 230, Carbohydrates 18 g, Fats 5 g, Proteins 27.5 g

Raspberry Lime Smoothie

Prep time 5 minutes/ Serves 2

Ingredients:

- 1 cup water
- 1 cup fresh or frozen raspberries
- 1 large frozen banana
- 2 tbsp fresh juice, lime
- 1 tsp oil, coconut
- 1 tsp agave

Directions:

1. In a blender put all ingredients and blend until smooth.
2. Take out and serve

Nutritional value per serving:

Calories 123, Carbohydrates 26.1 g, Fats 2.9 g, Proteins 1.5 g

Peppermint Monster Smoothie

Prep time 5 minutes/ Serves 1

Ingredients:

- 1 large frozen banana, peeled
- 1½ cups non-dairy milk
- A handful of fresh mint leaves, stems removed
- 1-2 handfuls spinach

Directions:

1. Add all ingredients in a blender and blend until smooth.
2. Take out and serve

Nutritional value per serving:

Calories 451, Carbohydrates 54.8 g, Fats 18.6 g, Proteins 18.4 g

Banana Green Smoothie

Prep time 5 minutes/ Serves 1

Ingredients:

- 1 cup coconut water
- ¾ cup plant-based milk
- ¼ tsp vanilla extract
- 1 heaping cup loosely packed spinach
- 2-3 cups frozen bananas, sliced

Directions:

1. Blend everything until smooth and serve.

Nutritional value per serving:

Calories 308, Carbohydrates 61 g, Fats 4.9 g, Proteins 10.2 g

Cinnamon Coffee Shake

Prep time 5 minutes/ Serves 2

Ingredients:

- 1 cup cooled coffee, regular or decaf
- ¼ cup almond or non-dairy milk
- A few pinches cinnamon
- 2 tbsp hemp seeds
- Splash vanilla extract
- 2 frozen bananas, sliced into coins
- Handful of ice

Directions:

2. Chill some coffee in a sealed container for a couple of hours (or overnight) before making this smoothie, or be ready to use more ice.
3. Add the non-dairy milk, cinnamon, vanilla, and hemp seeds to a blender and blend until smooth. Add the coffee and cut bananas and keep blending until smooth.
4. Add the ice and keep blending on high until there are no lumps remaining. Taste for sweetness and add your preferred plant-based sugar or sugar alternative.
5. Transfer to a glass and serve.

Nutritional value per serving:

Calories 73, Carbohydrates 11.7 g, Fats 2.2 g, Proteins 2.3 g

Orange Smoothie

Prep time 5 minutes/ Serves 2

Ingredients:

- 1 cup orange slices
- 1 cup mango chunks
- 1 cup strawberries, chopped
- 1 cup coconut water
- Pinch freshly grated ginger
- 1-2 cups crushed ice

Directions:

1. Place everything in a blender, blend, and serve.

Nutritional value per serving:

Calories 155, Carbohydrates 36.6 g, Fats 0.6 g, Proteins 2.9 g

Pumpkin Smoothie

Prep time 5 minutes/ Serves 2

Ingredients:

- 1 cup unsweetened non-dairy milk
- 2 medium bananas, peeled and cut into quarters and frozen
- 2 medjool dates, pitted
- 1 cup pumpkin puree, canned or fresh
- 2 cups ice cubes
- ¼ tsp cinnamon
- 2 tbsp ground flaxseeds
- 1 tsp pumpkin spice

Directions:

1. Blend all ingredients in a blender and serve.

Nutritional value per serving:

Calories 372, Carbohydrates 77.7 g, Fats 5.3 g, Proteins 9.2 g

Turmeric Smoothie

Prep time 5 minutes/ Serves 2

Ingredients:

- 2 cups non-dairy milk like coconut, almond
- 2 medium bananas, frozen
- 1 cup mango, frozen
- 1 tsp turmeric, ground grated, peeled
- 1 tsp fresh ginger, grated, peeled
- 1 tbsp chia seeds
- ¼ tsp vanilla extract
- ¼ tsp cinnamon, ground
- 1 pinch pepper, ground

Directions:

1. Blend all ingredients in a blender and serve

Nutritional value per serving:

Calories 264, Carbohydrates 51 g, Fats 4.4 g, Proteins 9.2 g

Veggie Smoothie

Prep time 10 minutes/ Serves 1

Ingredients:

- 1 stalk celery
- 1 carrot peeled and roughly chopped
- ½ cup broccoli sprouts
- 1 cup kale, chopped
- ½ cup curly parsley
- ½ tomato roughly chopped
- ½ avocado
- 1 banana
- ½ green apple
- ½ cup non-dairy milk
- 1 tbsp chia seeds
- 1 tbsp flaxseeds

Directions:

2. Place all ingredients in a blender.
3. Blend until smooth. Serve immediately.

Nutritional value per serving:

Calories 372, Carbohydrates 18 g, Fats 16 g, Proteins 7 g

Conclusion

Thank you for getting to the end of this book.

Choosing the perfect diet plan can be confusing thanks to the variety of diet plans available these days. Irrespective of what diet plan you opt for, almost all nutritionists and dietitians across the globe recommend diet plans that limit processed foods and that are based more on whole and fresh foods. The Plant-Based Diet is based on these universally preferred foods.

The whole-food plant-based diet plan is more flexible and understanding than other diets, too. It is mostly comprised of plant-based foods, but you can also have some animal-based products. The extent of animal-based foods in your diet plan depends on your personal choice to entirely not eat them or to consume them in moderation. In general, the more of your meals that are plant-based, the more beneficial the diet will be for you.

The primary focus of a plant-based, whole-food diet plan is to minimize the intake of processed foods as much as possible and consume more plant-based, whole natural foods that are proven to be beneficial for not only improving your health but also stimulating effective weight loss.

As you start your plant-based diet journey, use this guide to help you through and you can be sure that you be successful.

CPSIA information can be obtained
at www.ICGtesting.com
Printed in the USA
LVHW030149021120
670428LV00006B/175